GUIDE TO REPROCESSING OF HEMODIALYZERS

DEVELOPMENTS IN NEPHROLOGY

Cheigh, J.S., Stenzel, K.H., Rubin, A.L., eds.: Manual of Clinical Nephrology of the Rogosin Kidney Center. 1981. ISBN 90-247-2397-3.
Nolph, K.D., ed.: Peritoneal Dialysis. 1981. ISBN 90-247-2477-5.
Gruskin, A.B. and Norman, M.E., eds.: Pediatric Nephrology. 1981. ISBN 90-247-2514-3.
Schück, O., ed.: Examination of the Kidney Function, 1981. ISBN 0-89838-565-2.
Strauss, J., ed.: Hypertension, Fluid-Electrolytes and Tubulopathies in Pediatric Nephrology. 1981. ISBN 90-247-2633-6.
Strauss, J., ed.: Neonatal Kidney and Fluid-Electrolytes, 1983. ISBN 0-89838-575-X.
Strauss, J., ed.: Acute Renal Disorders and Renal Emergencies. 1984. ISBN 0-89838-663-2.
Didio, L.J.A. and Motta, P.M., eds.: Basic, Clinical and Surgical Nephrology. 1985. ISBN 0-89838-698-5.
Friedman, E.A. and Peterson, C.M., eds.: Diabetic Nephropathy: Strategy for Therapy. 1985. ISBN 0-89838-735-3.
Dzurik, R., Lichardus, B. and Guder, W., eds.: Kidney Metabolism and Function, 1985. ISBN 0-89838-749-3.
Strauss, J., ed.: Homeostasis, Nephrotoxicity, and Renal Anomalies in the Newborn. 1985. ISBN 0-89838-766-3.

GUIDE TO REPROCESSING OF HEMODIALYZERS

edited by

NORMAN DEANE
ROBERT J. WINEMAN
JAMES A. BEMIS
MANHATTAN KIDNEY CENTER

MARTINUS NIJHOFF PUBLISHING
A MEMBER OF THE KLUWER ACADEMIC PUBLISHERS GROUP
BOSTON   DORDRECHT   LANCASTER

Distributors

for the United States and Canada: Kluwer Academic Publishers, 101 Philip Drive, Norwell, MA 02061, USA

for the UK and Ireland: Kluwer Academic Publishers, MTP Press Limited, Falcon House, Queen Square, Lancaster LA1 1RN, UK

for all other countries: Kluwer Academic Publishers Group, Distribution Centre, P.O. Box 322, 3300 AH Dordrecht, The Netherlands

Library of Congress Cataloging-in-Publication Data

Guide to reprocessing of hemodialyzers.

(Developments in nephrology)
Includes index.
1. Hemodialysis—Equipment and supplies. 2. Artificial kidney—Maintenance and repair. I. Deane, Norman, 1921– . II. Wineman, Robert J. III. Bemis, James A. IV. Series. [DNLM: 1. Hemodialysis—instrumentation. W1 DE998EB/WJ 378 G946]
RC901.7.H45G85 1986   617'.461059   86-828
ISBN-13: 978-1-4612-9423-8   e-ISBN-13: 978-1-4613-2313-6
DOI: 10.1007/978-1-4613-2313-6

Copyright © 1986 by Martinus Nijhoff Publishing
Softcover reprint of the hardcover 1st edition 1986

To
Ronald E. Easterling, M.D.
1932–1986

CONTENTS

CONTRIBUTING AUTHORS

James A. Bemis, Ph.D.
Staff Scientist
Manhattan Kidney Center
40 East 30 Street
New York, New York 10016, USA

Ira C. Berman, M.D.
Staff Physician
Manhattan Kidney Center
40 East 30 Street
New York, New York 10016, USA

Lee A. Bland
Research Sanitarian
Nosocomial Infections Laboratory
    Branch
Hospital Infections Program
Center for Infectious Diseases
Centers for Disease Control
Atlanta, Georgia 30333, USA

Felix P. Brunner, M.D.
Privatdozent, Department of
    Medicine
University of Basel, Kantonsspital
CH-4031 Basel, Switzerland

Hans O.A. Brynger, M.D.
Associate Professor of Surgery
Department of Surgery I
Sahlgrens Hospital
S-41345 Gothenburg, Sweden

Sabri Challah, M.D.
Director, EDTA Registry
St. Thomas' Hospital
London, SE1 7EH
United Kingdom

Dennis E. Chenoweth, M.D., Ph.D.
Clinical Investigator
Veterans Administration Medical
    Center and
Associate Professor of Pathology
University of California, San Diego
3350 La Jolla Village Drive
San Diego, California 92161, USA

Norman Deane, M.D.
Medical Director
Manhattan Kidney Center
40 East 30 Street
New York, New York 10016, USA

Ronald E. Easterling, M.D.*
1490 Country View Lane
Flint, Michigan 48504, USA

W. Fassbinder, M.D.
Privatdozent
Abteilung fur Nephrologie
Lentrum Innere Medizin
Klinikum d. J.W. Goethe Universitat
Theodor-Stern-Kai 7
D-6000 Frankfurt Am Main 70, FRG

Martin S. Favero, Ph.D.
Chief, Nosocomial Infections
    Laboratory Branch
Hospital Infections Program
Center for Infectious Diseases
Centers for Disease Control
Atlanta, Georgia 30333, USA

T.H.J. Goodship, M.R.C.P.
Research Associate
Department of Medicine
University of Newcastle upon Tyne
Newcastle upon Tyne, NW2 4HH
United Kingdom

Frank A. Gotch, M.D.
Medical Director
Hemodialysis Treatment and
    Research Center
Franklin Hospital
Castro and Duboce
San Francisco, California 94114, USA

Lee W. Henderson, M.D.
Associate Chief of Staff for
    Research and Development
Veterans Administration Medical
    Center and
Professor of Medicine
University of California, San Diego
3350 La Jolla Village Drive
San Diego, California 92161, USA

Nicholas A. Hoenich, Ph.D.
Lecturer in Clinical Science
Department of Medicine
University of Newcastle upon Tyne
Newcastle upon Tyne, NE2 4HH
United Kingdom

Karl M. Koch, M.D.
Professor of Medicine
Medizinische Hochschule Hannover
Konstanty-Gutschow Strasse 8
D-3000 Hannover 61, FRG

Nathan W. Levin, M.D., F.A.C.P.
Clinical Professor
Department of Internal Medicine
University of Michigan, Ann Arbor, and
Henry Ford Hospital
2799 West Grand Boulevard
Detroit, Michigan 48202, USA

David L. Maude, M.D.
Associate Medical Director
Manhattan Kidney Center
40 East 30 Street
New York, New York 10016, USA

Anthony Messana
Technical Supervisor
Fairlane Health Services Corporation and
Henry Ford Hospital
2799 West Grand Boulevard
Detroit, Michigan 48202, USA

Mary Ann Miller-Messana
Staff Educator
Fairlane Health Services Corporation and
Henry Ford Hospital
2799 West Grand Boulevard
Detroit, Michigan 48202, USA

David A. Ogden, M.D., F.A.C.P.
Chief, Renal Section and
Professor of Medicine
University of Arizona
College of Medicine
Tucson, Arizona 85724, USA

R. Oules
Centre Hospitalier Regional et
Universitaire de Nimes
Nimes, France

S. Ringoir, M.D., Ph.D.
Professor of Medicine
Director of Renal Division
University of Gent
Gent, Belgium

---

* *Deceased.*

Neville H. Selwood, Ph.D.
Top Grade Scientific Officer
UK Transplant Service
Southmead Hospital
Bristol, BS10 5ND
United Kingdom

Michael K. Ward, F.R.C.P.
Senior Lecturer
Department of Medicine
University of Newcastle upon Tyne
Newcastle upon Tyne, NE2 4HH
United Kingdom

Robert J. Wineman, Ph.D.
Director, Special Projects
Manhattan Kidney Center
40 East 30 Street
New York, New York 10016, USA

Antony J. Wing, M.D., D.M., F.R.C.P.
Consulting Physician
St. Thomas' Hospital
London, SE1 7EH
United Kingdom

PREFACE

The purpose of this book is to provide information for the nephrologist to gain a perspective on the medical, scientific, and technical aspects of reprocessing of hemodialyzers. The book is also designed to serve the needs of the associated medical, nursing, and technical staffs of dialysis facilities for data on reuse of hemodialyzers. As an information source, the book will prove to be useful for those who may be considering reprocessing of dialyzers, as well as persons who are currently involved in this aspect of the practice of nephrology.

We have focused on the clinical and technological aspects of hemodialyzer reprocessing and have not dealt with socioeconomic considerations. We do wish to share with physicians performing hemodialysis several observations we have made as a result of assembling this volume. We believe that hemodialyzer reuse has had a beneficial impact on the quality of care for hemodialysis patients in consideration of the following factors. There is an increased awareness of membrane biocompatibility issues that has been brought to the forefront with the application of reuse. Utilization of hemodialyzer reprocessing has enabled nephrologists to compare the effect of various measures on biocompatibility when the patient is exposed to either a new or a reprocessed device. Previously, few readily available comparisons existed.

In the practice of dialysis, water quality has always been of considerable importance. With the advent of widespread hemodialyzer reprocessing, the issues of water bacteriology and water quality have become more prominent.

Generally the result has been an improvement in the quality of water used both for dialysis as well as for reprocessing.

The existence of reprocessing techniques enabled data to be generated that have permitted manufacturers to become aware of possible adverse effects of residua in new dialyzers. This has stimulated the industry to reduce such residues in new dialyzers, thus improving the biocompatibility of the products marketed.

Availability of reuse technology has made the development and marketing of more effective and costly dialyzers practical. Without reprocessing, the likelihood of use of larger high-flux dialyzers or hemofilters in the tight economy prevalent in the United States would be very unlikly. The application of reprocessing enables nephrologists to consider use of the more expensive devices for shorter-time therapy while remaining within today's imposed economic constraints.

Increased awareness of the concepts of quality control and quality assurance, which has been stimulated by dialyzer reprocessing, also applies to the entire treatment of hemodialysis and has had beneficial effects upon quality of care.

We gratefully acknowledge the contributions of all of our distinguished colleagues, whose work was essential in creating this volume. We also wish to acknowledge the dedication and hard work of our staff: Sheila Valz, Helen Szterenfeld, and Julie McDonagh.

GUIDE FOR REPROCESSING OF HEMODIALYZERS

1. EVOLUTION OF HEMODIALYZER REPROCESSING

NORMAN DEANE
IRA C. BERMAN

The practice of reuse of hemodialyzers is now approximately 25 years old. Although common in early dialysis facilities and home programs because of major economic restraints and, in some situations convenience, reuse practice declined in the United States when federal funding for hemodialysis became available. Interest in dialyzer reuse has been rekindled in the nephrology community in the last few years. According to two recent surveys the majority of facilities in this country are involved in dialyzer reuse. The acceptance of reuse has probably occurred for several reasons: (a) repeated demonstration of its safety when proper techniques are followed; (b) trends toward standardization of techniques, which has facilitated construction of several automated reuse systems; (c) the domination of the dialyzer market by the hollow-fiber dialyzer, which is particularly suited to reuse methods; and (d) current or anticipated future economic pressures sensed by directors of dialysis facilities.

HISTORY OF TECHNICAL EXPERIENCE

Initial motivations for reuse were economic and convenience. Shaldon [1] began reusing the Kolff twin-coil kidney in 1960 for daily dialysis of acute renal failure patients to make the most of his hospital's budget for disposable dialyzers. An additional advantage of his reuse procedure was that the patient's own blood was stored in the dialyzer, decreasing the need for outside blood sources to prime this large volume dialyzer. Refrigeration[1] was used to

3

inhibit bacterial growth; however, if the dialyzers were not reused within 24 h, febrile reactions occurred due to growth of cold-resistant bacteria[2].

To help the home hemodialysis patient avoid the arduous task of reconstructing the Kiil dialyzer, Pollard et al. [2] developed a technique to reuse the dialyzer and blood tubing. The methodology involved the basic steps of reprocessing that are currently used either in manual or automated reprocessing systems: (a) rinsing, (b) cleaning, (c) sterilization or disinfection, and (d) preparation for subsequent use. The technique developed by Pollard and coworkers involved cleaning the dialyzer with sodium hypochlorite and chemical sterilization with 1.5% formaldehyde. Their rationale for the use of a cleaning agent was to remove white blood cells and fibrin deposits left in the dialyzer following rinsing. These residual blood components might affect dialyzer performance and play a role in pyrogenic reactions that Shaldon had found to occur in his reuse procedure. Additionally, Pollard et al. found that sodium hypochlorite was inappropriate as a sterilizing agent[3], in that prolonged dialyzer exposure led to an unacceptably high incidence of membrane leakage. On the other hand, formaldehyde did not appear to have any deleterious effect on the dialyzer membranes. Testing for residual formaldehyde in the dialyzer at the time of subsequent usage was found to be most easily performed using CLINITEST® tablets. The sensitivity of the test was 1 part formaldehyde to 40,000 parts of saline. Although satisfactory as a screening procedure, this test was later found to be too insensitive for measuring low concentrations of residual formaldehyde which have been targeted.

With the advent of newer coil dialyzers containing lower priming volumes, blood priming prior to dialysis became unnecessary. Coil dialysis became quite popular because of the ease of technical set up compared with the Kiil. However, many facilities that desired to use coil dialyzers in the late 1960s faced economic pressures to reuse the dialyzers that were originally designed by the manufacturers as disposable items. In the days of dialysis committees, limited budgets could be stretched to treat more patients by reusing the coils. Satisfactory results were initially reported reusing coil dialyzers chemically sterilized and stored with formaldehyde (0.83%—4.0%), benzalkonium chloride (1:750) with refrigeration at 4°C [3, 4], and sterile water stored in the blood compartment while the entire dialyzer was kept immersed in a refrigerated 27% saline solution [5]. These methods generally involved rinsing the blood compartment of the dialyzer prior to storage with sterile water or saline to remove residual blood components.

By the early 1970s reuse methods were adapted to the disposable parallel plate dialyzers [6—9]. Since this dialyzer has a rigid internal support structure, rinsing of blood components from the dialyzer could be accomplished using fluid pressure in both the blood compartments and dialysate compartment with less risk of rupturing the membrane as compared with a coil dialyzer. Increasing fluid pressure during rinsing would theoretically displace more blood components from the dialysis membrane than low-pressure rinsing. Parallel plate dialyzers could also be stored by sealing off both the blood and dialysate compartments after the sterilant was introduced, thus closing the system to bacterial contamination during storage.

The hollow-fiber kidney first became commercially available in 1970 [10] and by 1972 the first report of reuse was published [11]. The hollow-fiber dialyzer soon proved to be particularly suited to reuse for several reasons.

The geometric rigidity of the individual hollow fibers provided a means to improve mechanical rinsing of the dialyzer. Water pressure could be applied from the dialysis compartment to the outside of the cylindrically shaped hollow fibers resulting in reverse ultrafiltration, helping to dislodge fibrin and blood components from the interior or blood compartment of the hollow fibers [12].

The rigid geometry of the hollow fiber also provided, through a measurement of cell volume, a practical, on-line estimate of membrane area and hence dialyzer function. Cell volume, also called fiber bundle volume (FBV), proved to be a rapid, reproducible measurement. In contrast, since it is not possible to determine, on-line, the functioning surface area of a coil or plate dialyzer with multiple use, function of these types of dialyzers could only be determined from clearance measurements [13]. This has led to the nearly universal adoption of the hollow-fiber dialyzer for reuse, since its residual function can be verified easily after each treatment.

REUSE: CLINICAL EXPERIENCE

Clinical experience with multiple use of hemodialyzers began in 1964 with coil dialyzers [1]. Since that time, the multiple-use technique has been applied to all types of dialyzers. Although variations in the techniques of multiple use at one time were considerable, there has been some standardization of the process in the last few years. With repeated demonstration of the safety of the procedure along with satisfactory clinical results, there has been widespread acceptance of hemodialyzer reuse in the United States. Although survey data indicated that in 1978 only 17.2% of United States ESRD facilities were involved in dialyzer reprocessing [14], that figure had grown to over 51% of the facilities by 1984 [15].

Large-scale clinical data were not available until the completion of the surveys by the European Dialysis and Transplant Association (EDTA) in 1976 [16, 17] and 1977 [18]. According to these surveys, patients treated with reused dialyzers survived as long or longer than patients treated with single-use dialyzers (table 1-1) [19]. Unfortunately, these are the only data on survival statistics for patients treated with reused dialyzers. Concerning the immediate treatment setting, a report from the National Workshop on the Reuse of Consumables in Hemodialysis [20] concluded that "when appropriate reprocessing standards are followed there is negligible or no risk of mortality."

Table 1-1. Annual mortality in dialysis centers

| | Patient (Number) | | Mortality (%) | | |
	Reusing	Not reusing	Reusing	Not reusing	p
Five European countries EDTA Registry, 1976	591	3491	6.8	8.8	0.057
Five European countries EDTA Registry, 1977					
Ages 35−44	175	749	1.2	8.8	0.0001
Ages 45−54	242	1021	5.0	5.3	0.40
United Kingdom	98	130	6.5	15.6	0.22

Reproduced with permission from Lowrie Hakim [19].

Far more information is available on the morbidity associated with dialyzer reuse as compared with single use. The available data include studies showing improvement in certain aspects of the dialysis treatment when a reprocessed rather than a new dialyzer is used.

The patient with uremia receiving hemodialysis treatment has reduced immunologic competence and is, at the same time, subjected to the hazards of repeated extracorporeal circulation. This combination entails a serious risk of infectious complication if meticulous technique is not employed. There is, however, no indication that multiple use has increased the risk of infectious complications when formaldehyde in an appropriate concentration and with a suitable technique has been employed as the antimicrobial agent [21]. Following outbreaks of waterborne atypical mycobacteria infections in two Louisiana dialysis facilities involved in reprocessing with 2% formaldehyde, the Centers for Disease Control has recommended [22] that a higher concentration (4%) be used. This level of formaldehyde has been demonstrated to be effective against these organisms [23, 24]. Likewise, less effective sterilants such as benzalkonium chloride [5, 25] and 27% sodium chloride [26, 27] have been dropped from reuse protocols.

It has been shown that the incidence of hepatitis is no greater in units that reuse dialyzers than in units that practice single use of dialyzers [28]. To reduce the risks of further blood handling, most dialysis facilities involved in reuse do not reprocess dialyzers of hepatitis-positive patients. However, there is no definitive contraindication to reprocessing dialyzers of hepatitis-positive patients. Epidemiologic considerations would suggest that hepatitis-positive and -negative dialyzers be reprocessed in separate areas.

Hospitalization rates are an important way to assess morbidity, yet limited data are available comparing such statistics for patients receiving treatment with reused dialyzers as opposed to single-use dialyzers. Kant and associates [29] analyzed the rates of hospitalization of these groups as an index of the

Table 1-2. Frequency of hospitalization in 27 ESRD patients

	Single use (320 pt mos)	Multiple-use unit (334 pt mos)
Days of hospitalization per patient month Not Related to Dialysis	0.43	0.48
Days of hospitalization per patient month Related to Dialysis	0.89	0.48

Data from Kant et al. [29].

morbidity of hemodialysis treatment. They followed 27 patients treated for 320 and 334 patient months, respectively, in separate dialysis facilities that practiced single use and reuse. They observed that certain symptoms occurred with greater frequency in patients receiving first-use dialyzers as opposed to patients receiving dialysis treatment with reused dialyzers. Such complications included fever, sweating, chest pains, respiratory distress, hypotension, nausea, and vomiting. The rates of hospitalization for dialysis-related problems were also significantly higher for patients on single-use dialysis (table 1-2).

A constellation of symptoms typical of an allergic reaction has been observed to occur occasionally on treatment with a new dialyzer. Appropriately termed the "new dialyzer" syndrome [30], it is characterized by back or chest pain, respiratory distress with or without frank wheezing, and chills or fever occurring shortly after the start of dialysis. Urticaria has also been observed. Symptoms may be mild, but occasionally they resemble a severe anaphylactic reaction.

Levin et al. [31], in a well-designed double-blind study comparing therapy with new and reused hollow-fiber dialyzers, also found that the incidence of back and chest pain was significantly greater when a new dialyzer was used. In their study, neither staff nor patient was aware of which dialyzer was being used, as it was contained in an opaque box (figures 1-1 and 1-2).

Proponents of dialyzer reuse feel that these clinical observations and studies indicate that a reused dialyzer is more biocompatible than a new one. In support of this are some observations on white blood cell and serologic alterations that take place during a hemodialysis treatment. Kaplow and Goffinet [32] first showed that a transient neutropenia accompanied initiation of hemodialysis with the twin-coil dialyzer. This observation was confirmed by Gral et al. [33] 1979 and extended to the hollow-fiber and Kiil dialyzers. Savdie et al. [34] later demonstrated that the neutropenic response was more severe with a new hollow-fiber dialyzer than with reused dialyzers. More recently, Lowrie and Hakim [19] have shown that cellophane and CUPROPHAN® dialyzers exhibit a greater reduction of the white blood cell

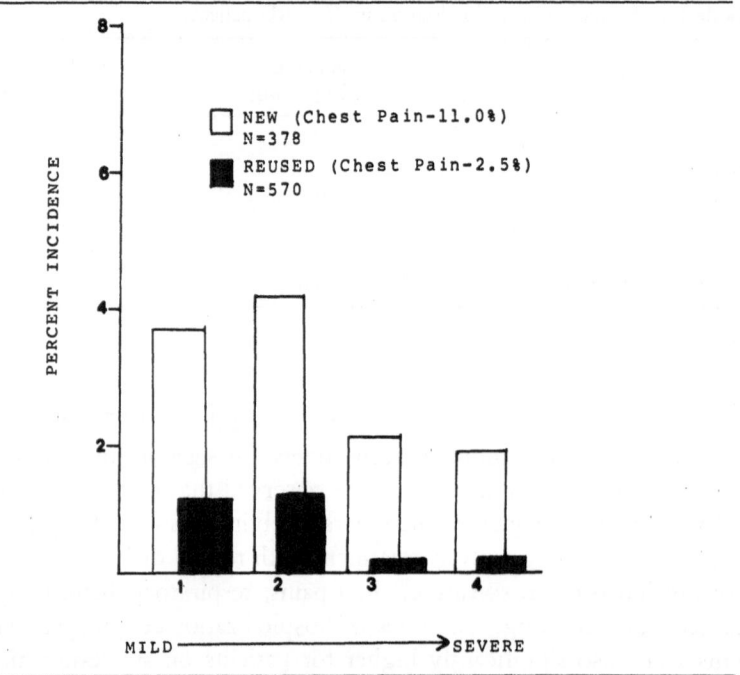

Figure 1-1. The incidence of chest pain is significantly greater with new dialyzers ($p = 0.013$). Reproduced, with permission, from Bok et al. [31].

count and serum complement when new as opposed to reused (figures 1-3 and 1-4). Stroncek et al. [35] have shown that formaldehyde contributes to changes in dialyzer membranes, which may enhance their biocompatibility similar to the process that occurs when heart valves are treated with formaldehyde.

At least two mechanisms may be involved: (a) Residual materials left in the dialyzer from the manufacturing process may leach out during use. Studies performed at the Centers for Disease Control (CDC), US Public Health Service, have demonstrated significant release of limulus amebocyte lysate (LAL)-active material from the blood and dialysate compartments of a new dialyzer following a 16-h soak [36]. The leaching rate of LAL-active material from the blood compartment of two new dialyzers was tested and shown to decrease as the dialyzers were flushed on subsequent days. (b) Interaction of humoral or formed elements of the blood with the dialyzer membrane may result in release of pharmacologically active substances which may account for pyrogenic reactions or anaphylactic phenomena.

Repeated use and reprocessing of the dialyzer may reduce both of these deleterious effects. There will be less residue from the manufacturing process after the initial use. Further, after the initial protein—membrane interaction has taken place, enhanced biocompatibility of the dialyzer should be in-

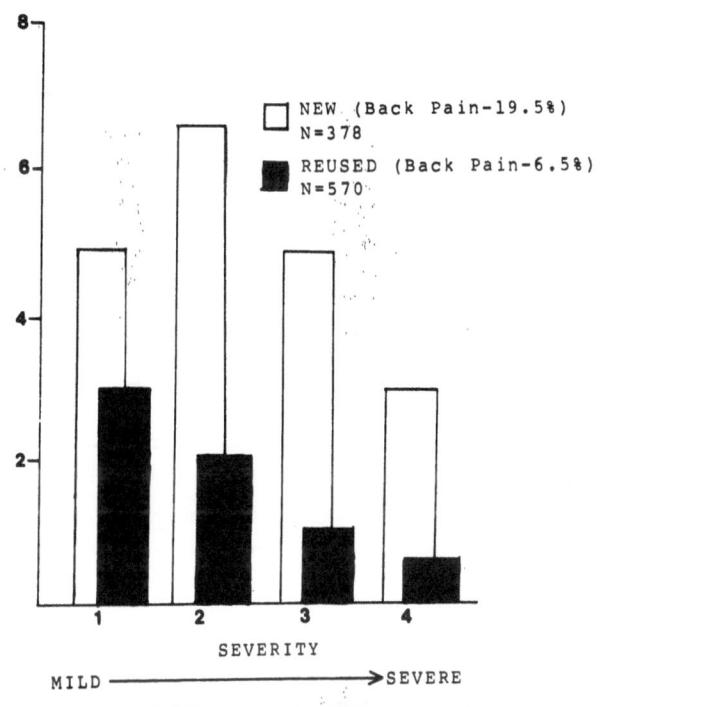

Figure 1-2. The incidence of back pain is significantly greater with new dialyzers ($p = 0.0005$). Reproduced, with permission, from Bok et al. [31].

creased.

Patient exposure to residual formaldehyde left in the dialyzer following the full reuse procedure can result in the production of antibodies to the red blood cell N-antigen. This so called anti-N-like antibody, first identified by Howell and Perkins [37] in 1972, has been implicated in exacerbating anemia [38]. (Refer to chapter 9 for a full discussion of anti-N-like antibodies.) Rarely, patients have been reported to experience burning at the site of infusion at the start of dialysis, attributable to residual formaldehyde in the dialyzer. This has occurred despite negative CLINITEST® results for formaldehyde presence [39]. The authors are not aware of any reports of accidental infusions of formaldehyde to patients from any unflushed or improperly prepared, reprocessed dialyzers. Such incidents should not occur with proper quality control measures.

A potential exists for inadequate or underdialysis if treatments are performed with reused dialyzers that have poor clearances. Since measuring clearances is too cumbersome for routine use, it is fortunate that a correlation between changes in cell volume (fiber bundle volume) of hollow-fiber dialyzers and changes in clearnaces of small solutes has been developed (see figure 3-3 of chapter 3) [40]. Using fiber bundle volume measurements, one can

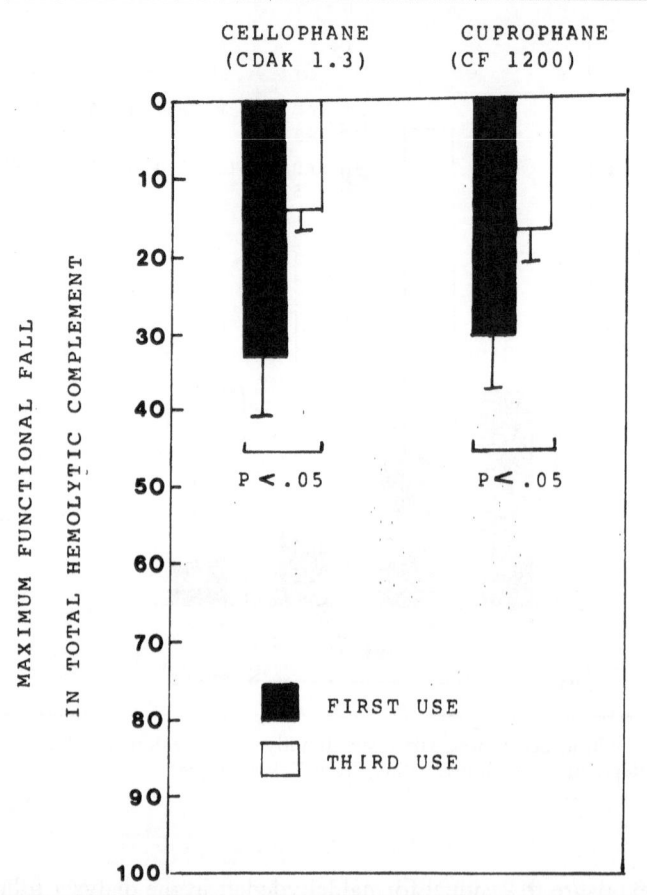

Figure 1-3. Fractional decrease in serum complement with new and reused hollow-fiber dialyzers. Reproduced, with permission, from Lowrie and Hakim [19].

reject dialyzers (for continued use) that are below a critical volume measurement. Present recommendations are to reject dialyzers that have less than 80% of their initial priming volume [41]. This seems to correlate with approximately a 10% decrease in urea clearance of the dialyzer. By monitoring fiber bundle volume along with other parameters commonly used to ascertain adequacy of dialysis, the potential for undertreatment of an individual patient should be no different than with single-use dialyzers. (Refer to chapter 3 for further information on dialyzer transport with reuse.)

In summary, dialyzer reuse has now been practiced for over 20 years and applied to thousands of patients and probably hundreds of thousands or millions of dialysis treatments. Although further study of the long-term effects of dialyzer reuse on patient outcome is warranted, available data do not suggest any increased risk of mortality or major morbidity. In fact, reuse may have some salutary effects on the course of a dialysis treatment. The

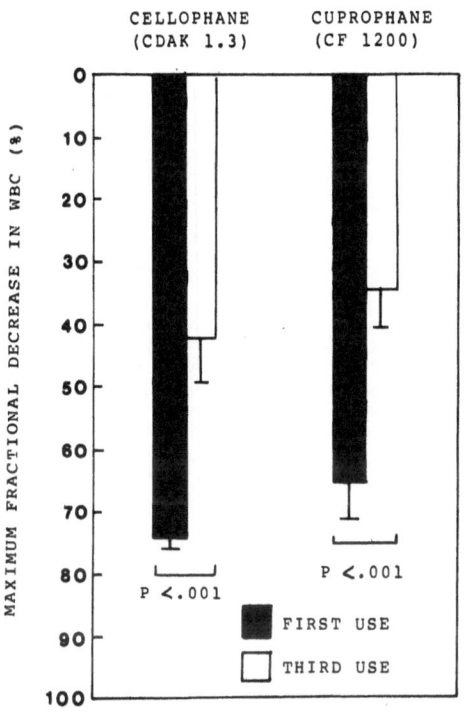

Figure 1-4. Fractional decrease in white blood count with new and reused hollow-fiber dialyzers. Reproduced, with permission, from Lowrie and Hakim [19].

care with which the reprocessing procedure is applied is crucial for satisfactory clinical results. Where attention to detail slackens or the method is inadequate, complications may be encountered.

PRESENT STATUS OF HEMODIALYZER REUSE IN THE UNITED STATES

In the last five years there has been a rekindling of interest in dialyzer reuse in the United States. To gain insight into current reuse practices, a survey was conducted by the National Nephrology Foundation in 1984 [15]. The results of this survey were reported at the AAMI conference on hemodialyzer reuse in 1984. A similar survey was conducted by the Renal Physicians Association in 1978 [14]. An interim survey was also conducted in 1981, but never reported.

In the 1984 survey, data were gathered from 51.5% of approved United States ESRD suppliers and (some) 635 facilities responded to 1233 inquiries. Response rate in 1978 was higher at 73.0%. In the 1984 survey, 55.6% of patients were being treated with multiple usage of dialyzers, whereas only 16.0% were treated in the same fashion in 1978 (table 1-3). Similar statistics were observed for reuse practices by facility: 51.4% of surveyed facilities

12

Table 1-3. Patient distribution on reused dialyzers 1978[1] vs 1984.

	In-center		Home		Totals	
	1978	1984	1978	1984	1978	1984
Number of hemodialysis patients	27,173	33,386	4,715	2,832	31,888	36,218
Number of patients treated with multiple usage of dialyzers	4,341	18,569	656	89	4,997	18,658
Percent of patients treated with multiple usage of dialyzers	16.0	55.6	13.9	3.1	15.7	51.5
Percent of patients treated by single usage of dialyzers	84.0	44.4	86.1	96.9	84.3	48.5

Table 1-4. Incidence of multiple usage of dialyzers according to ESRD supplier activity 1978[1] vs 1984.

Number of patients per facility (in-center and home)	Facilities employing multiple usage				Facilities employing single usage			
	Number		%		Number		%	
	1978	1984	1978	1984	1978	1984	1978	1984
1–30	28	71	11.2	38.0	250	116	89.9	62.0
31–60	43	108	22.8	52.2	145	99	77.2	47.8
61–100	22	77	20.5	58.3	85	55	79.5	32.6
100	14	60	28.5	67.4	35	29	71.5	32.6
Totals	107	316	17.2	51.4	515	299	82.8	48.6

Table 1-5. Distribution of dialyzer types for reused and single-use dialyzers 1978 or 1984.

	Multiple usage		Single Usage	
	1978	1984	1978	1984
Hollow fiber (%)	65.2	99.4	36.7	78.7
Parallel plate (%)	23.6	0.5	15.5	20.5
Coil (%)	11.2	0.1	47.8	0.8
Totals	100.0	100.0	100.0	100.0

practiced multiple usage of hemodialyzers in 1984 as compared with only 17.2% in 1978 (table 1-4). A general trend was present during both surveys for larger centers to be more commonly involved in reuse. However, even facilities with less than 31 patients had a significant minority (38%) involved in reuse during 1984.

Near universal selection of the hollow-fiber dialyzer as the unit of choice for reuse has occurred (table 1-5). However, even facilities not involved in multiple usage showed a particular preference for hollow-fiber dialyzers (78.7% of patients on single used dialyzers), whereas coil dialyzers are rarely being used for hemodialysis treatments in the United States.

Automation has also taken a major foothold in reprocessing (see chapter 11). Already, 39.5% of facilities involved in reuse of dialyzers have some automated equipment, whereas 58% of facilities are using manual reprocessing alone. According to the survey, it did not appear that automation provided a statistical advantage in the number of uses obtained per dialyzer (automated 9.12 ± 3.77 vs manual 8.19 ± 3.28). Using cleaning agents such as sodium hypochlorite, peroxide, or peroxyacetic acid in the reprocessing procedure also did not appear to improve the number of uses obtained per dialyzer as compared with rinsing alone.

In summary, dialyzer reuse has become a thoroughly accepted methodology in end-stage renal disease. Although the impetus for reuse is largely economic, the main reason for its growth has been the repeated demonstration that the procedure is safe and effective when performed properly. Although dialyzer reuse is practiced by the majority of ESRD facilities in the United States, additional studies are warranted concerning its impact on the morbidity and mortality of the patient population.

NOTES

[1]Cold storage refers to refrigerated storage usually around 4°C.

[2]Cold bacteria refers to bacteria that may continue to grow during refrigeration, such as pseudomonas and atypical mycobacteria.

[3]Although the terms disinfection and sterilization or disinfecting agent and sterilizing agent may be used interchangeably in this chapter, they actually are not equivalent. Although the term sterilization has been commonly applied to the procedure of adding a chemical agent to the dialyzer for storage, the proper technical

term is disinfection. "Sterilization is defined as a procedure effected by either physical or chemical agents that results in the total destruction of micro-organism including highly resistant bacterial spores." "Disinfection is defined as a process that is generally less lethal than sterilization and results in the elimination of most recognized pathogens but not necessarily the more resistant micro-organisms which include bacterial endo-spores" [22]. (Refer to chapter 4, "Microbiologic principles applied to reprocessing hemodialyzers".)

REFERENCES

1. Shaldon SH, Silva H, Rosen M: Technique for refrigerated coil preservation haemodialysis with femoral venous catheterization. Br Med J 2:411−413, 1964.
2. Pollard TL, Barnett BMS, Eschbach JW, Scribner BH: A technique for storage and multiple reuse of the Kiil dialyzer and blood tubing. Trans Am Soc Artif Intern Organs 13:24−28, 1967.
3. Johnson CE, Octaviano GN, Beirne GJ, Haynie GD, Burns RO: Cleaning, storage and repeated use of twin coil dialyzing units. JAMA 207:2087−2088, 1969.
4. Gottloib L, Servadio C: The routine re-utilization of 'disposable' coils for hemodialysis. Isr J Med Sci 8:79−80, 1972.
5. Bilinsky RT, Morris AJ: Hemodialysis coil reuse: a safe and economical new method. JAMA 218:1806−1808, 1971.
6. Fawsett KC, Mangles MD: Reuse of the Gambro Lundia 17-layer dialyzer. Dial Transplant 3:38−40, 1974.
7. Kramer P, Matthaei D, Go JG, Winckler K, Scheler F: Effect of blood factor deposits in reused dialysers on the dialysance of middle weight molecules. Proc Eur Dial Transplant Assoc 9:278−285, 1972.
8. Miach PJ, Evans SM, Wilcox AA, Dewborn JK: Reuse of a disposable dialyzer for home dialysis. Med J Aust 1:146−147, 1976.
9. Von Hartitizsch B, Hoenich NA, Kerr DNS: In vitro and in vivo assessment of the Rhone Poulene disposable dialyzer (type I B). Proc Eur Dial Transplant Assoc 8:401−404, 1971.
10. Gotch F, Lipps B, Weaver J, Brandes J, Rosin J, Sargent J, Oja P: Chronic hemodialysis with the hollow fiber artificial kidney (HFAK). Trans Am Soc Artif Intern Organs 15:87−96, 1969.
11. Eschbach JW, Vizzo JE: Evaluation of Dow hollow fiber artificial kidney. In: Proceedings of the 5th annual contractor's conference (Artificial Kidney Chronic Uremia Program, NIAMDD), 1972, pp 17−18.
12. Hirsch K, Grist G, Crouch T: A reuse method for the Cordis-Dow artificial kidney. Dial Transplant 5:76−78, 1976.
13. Deane N, Bemis JA: Multiple use of hemodialyzers. Manhattan Kidney Center. National Nephrology Foundation, New York, 1982, pp 28−29.
14. Deane N, Blagg C, Bower J, De Palma J, Gutch C, Kanter A, Odgen D, Sadler J, Siemsen, Teehan B, Sosin A: A survey of dialyzer reuse practice in the United States. Dial Transplant 7:1128−1130, 1978.
15. Deane N: A survey of dialyzer reuse practice in the United States 1984. In: Hemodialyzer reuse: issues and solutions. Association for Advancement of Medical Instrumentation, Arlington VA, 1985, pp 1−5.
16. Jacobs C, Brunner FP, Chantler C, Donckerwolcke RA, Gurland HJ, Hathaway RA, Selwood NJ, Wing AJ: Combined report on regular dialysis and transplantation in Europe VII. 1976. Proc Eur Dial Transplant Assoc 14:3:69, 1977.
17. Wing AJ, Brunner FP, Brynger H, Chantler C, Donckerwolcke RA, Gurland JJ, Jacobs C, Selwood NH: Mortality and morbidity of reusing dialyzers. Br Med J 2:853−855, 1978.
18. Wing AJ, Brunner FP, Brynger H, Chantler C, Donckerwolcke RA, Gurland HJ, Hathaway RA, Jacobs: Combined report on regular dialysis and transplantation in Europe, VIII. 1977. Proc Eur Dial Transplant Assoc 13:3−76, 1978.
19. Lowrie EG, Hakim RM: The effect on patient health of using reprocessed artificial kidneys. Proc Dial Transplant Forum 10:86−91, 1980.
20. Sadler J: Generally accepted conclusions from the national workshop on reuse of consumables in hemodialysis, appendix. In: Proceedings of national workshop on reuse of consumables in hemodialysis. Kidney Disease Coalition, Washington DC, 1982, P B-2.
21. Peterson NJ: Microbiologic hazards associated with reuse of hemodialyzers. In: National

workshop on reuse of consumables in hemodialysis. Kidney Disease Coalition, Washington DC, 1983, pp 119–134.

22. Favero MS: Distinguishing between high-level disinfection, reprocessing and sterilization in reuse of disposables. AAMI Technology Report no. 6–83, 1983, pp 19–23.
23. Center for Disease Control: Nontuberculous mycobacterial infections in hemodialysis patients: Louisiana. Morbid Mortal Week Rep 32:244–245, 1983.
24. Favero MS: Recommendations for water quality and sterilant concentrations. In: Deane N, Wineman RJ (eds) Seminar on reuse of hemodialyzers automated and manual methods. Manhattan Kidney Center. National Nephrology Foundation, New York, 1984, pp 28–36.
25. Mason RG, Zuker WH, Bilinsky RT, Shinoda BA, Sharp DE, Mohammad SF: Blood components deposited on used and reused dialysis membranes. Biomater Med Devices Artif Organs 4:333–358, 1976.
26. Gutch CF, Swanson JR, Ogden DA: Failure of dailysis concentrate as a bacterial agent. Proc Dial Transplant Forum 4:234–238, 1974.
27. Neff MS, Maloway M: Reuse of dialysis coils. JAMA 214:234–238, 1974.
28. Favero MS, Deane N, Leger RT, Sosin E: Effects of multiple use of dialyzers on hepatitis B incidence in patients and staff. JAMA 245:166–167, 1981.
29. Kant KS, Pollak VE, Cathey M, Goetz D, Berlin R, et al.: Multiple use of dialyzers: safety and efficacy. Kidney Int 19:728–738, 1981.
30. Ogden DA: New-dialyzer syndrome. N Engl J Med 302:1262–1263, 1980.
31. Bok DV, Pascual L, Herberger C, Sawyer R, Levin NW: Effect of multiple use of dialyzers on intradialytic symptoms. Proc Dial Transplant Forum 19:92–96, 1980.
32. Kaplow LS, Goffinet JA: Profound neutropenia during the early phase of hemodialysis. JAMA 203:1135, 1968.
33. Gral T, Schroth P, De Palma JR, Gordan A: Leukocyte dynamics with three types of hemodialyzers. Trans Am Soc Artif Inter Organs 15:45–49, 1969.
34. Savdie E, Bruce L, Vincent PC: Modified neutropenic response to re-used dialyzers in patients with chronic renal failure. Clin Nephrol 8:422–428, 1977.
35. Stroncek DF, Keshaviah P, Shaprio FL, Craddock PR: Effects of dialyzer re-use on fiber-induced complement (C) activation and hemodialysis (HD) granulocytopenia. Clin Res 29, 1981.
36. Petersen NJ, Carson LA, Favero MS: Bacterial endotoxin in new and reused hemodialyzers: a potential cause of endotoxemia. Trans Am Soc Artif Intern Organs 27:155–160, 1981.
37. Howell D, Perkins HA: Anti-N-like antibodies in the sera of patients undergoing chronic hemodialysis. Vox Sang 23:291–299, 1972.
38. Koch KM, Frei U, Fassbinder W: Hemolysis and anemia in anti-N-like antibody positive hemodialysis patients. Trans Am Soc Artif Intern Organs 24:709–713, 1978.
39. Reveillaud RJ, Deschamps A, Aubert P: Risks of I.V. administration of formaldehyde to hemodialyzed patients. Kidney Int 11:292–293, 1977.
40. Gotch FA: Mass transport in reused dialyzers. Proc Dial Transplant Forum 10:81–85, 1980.
41. AAMI proposed recommended practice for reuse of hemodialyzers (proposed) August 1985 Revision. Association for Advancement of Medical Instrumentation, Arlington VA, p 24.

2. REPROCESSING TECHNIQUES

NORMAN DEANE
DAVID L. MAUDE
JAMES A. BEMIS

Reuse of hemodialyzers has expanded from a seldom-used technique to one that is now practiced by the majority of providers of end-stage renal disease care in the United States [1, 2]. In 1984 the Association for the Advancement of Medical Instrumentation (AAMI), recognizing the widespread adoption of reprocessing procedures, drafted a "Recommended Practice for Reuse of Hemodialyzers," addressed to the physician responsible for reprocessing hemodialyzers either by manual or automated techniques [3]. The commercial availability, beginning in 1980–81, of automated reprocessing machines encouraged the spread of reuse, and automated devices are now used by 40% of the facilities practicing reuse in the United States [1].

This chapter surveys the literature of the last four years that deals with technical aspects of reprocessing hemodialyzers. Reviews of the earlier literature are available elsewhere [4–6]. We describe the component steps of reprocessing, and specific reuse procedures designed to preserve the mass transport capabilities and mechanical characteristics of the membrane, to minimize chemical contamination from reuse, and to insure the biological safety of the reprocessed hemodialyzer.

Because of the growing importance of "high-flux" hemodialyzers and hemodiafiltration, this survey includes reports dealing with the newer types of membrane devices, employing polyacrylonitrile, polysulfone, and polymethylmethacrylate fibers. We have not differentiated hemodialyzers from hemofilters and hemodiafilters because some devices may be used for more

Deane, Wineman, and Bemis (eds.): GUIDE TO REPROCESSING OF HEMODIALYZERS.
© 1986. Martinus Nijhoff Publishing. All rights reserved.

than one mode of therapy.

The purpose of this review is to identify elements of the reuse procedure that are the most important for improving the reuse process. In the survey conducted by Deane [1], the reported average number of dialyzer uses per facility varied widely, from two to 24 uses, indicating wide variation in reprocessing practices.

More important than merely increasing the number of reuses of each dialyzer is the quest for improved biocompatibility of the membrane. Most workers in the field would agree that we should not necessarily try to restore the membrane to its original condition, for evidence indicating that the reprocessed dialyzer may be more biocompatible than a new dialyzer continues to accumulate [7−9]. (See also chapters 1, 10, and 11.) It is possible that a specific protein coat left on the membrane after use produces a dialyzer that provides a better treatment for the patient [10]. Should this be true, efforts should be made to determine how best to reprocess each membrane type to provide the most favorable treatment for each patient.

COMPONENT STEPS IN REPROCESSING

The report from the National Workshop on Reuse of Consumables in Hemodialysis [6] described seven steps in the reprocessing procedure: (1) identification of the dialyzer, (2) rinsing, (3) cleaning (optional), (4) functional assessment, (5) sterilization (disinfection), (6) sterilant (disinfectant) removal, and (7) monitoring clinical care.

Step 2 deals with establishing procedures that insure that a given dialyzer remains associated with the same patient and recording dialyzer usage [11]. These are discussed by Levin et al. in chapter 5.

Step 7 involves: (1) monitoring monthly chemistries and other clinical data, (2) measuring clearances on a sampling basis, (3) monitoring patient symptoms, (4) discussions with patients, and (5) current awareness and application of the state of the art. These also are discussed elsewhere (see chapters 6−10).

Because certain procedures carried out prior to rinsing the dialyzer may have an impact on reprocessing, one additional step involving "prerinse procedures" should be added to this list. This step includes the specifics of heparinization of the patient, conditions for termination of dialysis, and details on handling the dialyzer prior to initiation of the rinsing step. Suboptimal conditions of heparin usage, for example, could produce clotting of half a dozen or so fibers in a hollow-fiber dialyzer, which for cosmetic reasons is taken as a basis for discarding the dialyzer [3, 11].

Rinsing

It is important that new dialyzers be rinsed thoroughly, for two reasons. Most allergic or hypersensitivity reactions, or the "new dialyzer" syndrome described by Ogden [12], could probably be avoided with more extensive rinsing than is recommended by the manufacturer. Klinkmann and Ivanovich [13] have described the materials being used for the production of cellulosic hollow-fiber dialyzers via the cuprammonium process:

Extrusion: aqueous copper solution, ammonia, glycerin, carbon disulfide
Core fluid: isopropyl myristate or other organic liquids
Regeneration: acid or alkaline baths
Core fluid removal: organic solvents
Ethylene oxide sterilization

Kuentz et al. [14] reported that 75% of hypersensitvity reactions observed in their survey of dialysis units in France resulted from failure to use the manufacturer's stated level of rinse-out procedures.

The second reason for rinsing new dialyzers is to obtain a reliable measure of total cell volume (TCV or FBV, fiber bundle volume), prior to first use. This permits comparison of the cell volume measured after reprocessing with that of the new dialyzer. The decrease should not exceed 20% of the original volume [6, 11, 15]. Because the variation in cell volume among dialyzers of the same type and lot number may be of the order of 10%−15% [4, 6], it is inappropriate to use a cell volume based on an average or random sampling of dialyzers, or the manufacturers stated value, to make this comparison.

Cleaning

The survey by Deane [1] showed that sodium hypochlorite and/or hydrogen peroxide were being used in over half of the centers in the United States that reprocessed hemodialyzers, with another 9% using other cleaning agents. Deane and Bemis [4] evaluated most of the cleaning agents which had been suggested for use with dialyzers, and found only sodium hypochlorite to be effective. The latter's reaction with cellulosic membranes is dependent on time, temperature, and concentration and its use should be closely monitored with dialyzers containing cellulosic materials.

Implicit with the utilization of a cleaning agent is the requirement that it be removed prior to storage of the dialyzer containing a sterilizing (disinfecting) agent. Additionally, the cleaning solution must not contain undesirable amounts of endotoxin.

Dialyzer assessment

After rinsing and cleaning, the dialyzer's functional characteristics should be assessed prior to sterilization and storage. The reuse workshop [6] dealt with the various measurements that may be employed: (1) cell volume, (2) ultrafiltration rate, (3) clearance, (4) pressure—flow rate (hydraulic resistance), and (5) direct observation. Some of these methods apply only to a specific type of dialyzer. Cell volume measurement, for example, is applicable only to hollow-fiber devices. Hollow fibers nominally have constant volume during use, but the aggregate volume may decrease with use when individual fibers become clogged with protein.

Preparation for use

Sterilants or disinfectants used for storing dialyzers must be removed and their concentrations reduced to negligible levels by flowing sterile saline on the blood side and use of flowing dialysate in the dialysate compartment before connecting the patient to the dialyzer [16]. Volumes of saline much larger than the cell volume or a saline recirculation technique are required because of binding of the disinfectant to materials in the dialyzer. With cellulosic membrances, Gotch and Keen [17] have shown that the polyurethane potting compound surrounding the fibers at the ends of the dialyzer binds formaldehyde and controls the kinetics of rinse out of this agent (see chapter 3). Similar considerations apply to membrane types and will determine in each instance which sterilizing agent can be most advantageously employed.

REUSE PROCEDURES

This review concentrates on hollow-fiber dialyzers, since 90% of the dialyzers sold throughout the world are of this type [13]. Reuse of plate dialyzers, often employed for home dialysis and for HBsAG-positive patients, continues to decrease, accounting for only 10% of the dialyzers used in the United States in 1984 [1]. Coil-type dialyzers, in this survey [1], accounted for less than 1% of the dialyzers in use.

Our discussion focuses on various membrane materials, recognizing of course that certain reuse procedures may apply to more than one type. This approach serves to emphasize that dialyzers, even of the same membrane material but from different manufacturers, may differ in details of production or construction and therefore in their requirements for optimal reprocessing.

The following materials will be considered: (1) cellulosic membranes: CUPROPHAN®—regenerated cellulose (cuprammonium cellulose); cuprammonium rayon—similar to CUPROPHAN®; new regenerated cellulose—similar to CUPROPHAN®; and cellulose acetate; (2) polyacrylonitrile (PAN); (3) polymethylmethacrylate (PMMA); (4) polysulfone (PS); (5) polypropylene (PP); and (6) polycarbonate (PC).

Although it is possible that the newer-type dialyzers can be reprocessed as easily as the older ones, it should be borne in mind that the structures and pore sizes of many of the newer membranes are quite different. For example, Sakai et al. [18] have calculated pore diameters of regenerated cellulose membranes to be 45–65 microns vs 55–125 microns for the synthetic polymeric type. Some membranes have wall thicknesses of only 5–10 microns, and may easily be damaged by the pressure-induced reverse ultrafiltration used to remove debris from the blood compartment of the dialyzer during reprocessing.

The procedures that follow were selected from the recent literature on the reprocessing of dialyzers. They were chosen to illustrate the variety of approaches being used, and were selected on the basis of the amount of detail which was provided by the various authors. We have included a description of our own reprocessing technique, not because we think it is better, but because of the specific detail that we can provide of each step.

Cellulosic membranes

Blagg [19] described dialyzer reprocessing procedures developed over a period of 14 years at the Northwest Kidney Center in Seattle for home dialysis patients. For cellulosic hollow-fiber dialyzers, their procedure is as follows:

1. The blood compartment is rinsed for 20 min at 1.2–1.5 liters/min.
2. Volume test the dialyzer.
3. Rinse the blood compartment with 0.5 liter of 1.5% formaldehyde and clamp. After 2 h, the dialysate side is flushed with 1.5% formaldehyde (HCHO) and the dialyzer is stored until the next use.
4. Preparation for use consists of a 1-liter saline rinse of the blood compartment, clamping the lines for 20 min, and then rinsing with 0.5 liter saline. Finally, the dialysate side is rinsed with saline before testing the dialyzer for residual HCHO.

Hollow-fiber dialyzers are typically used three times.

The storage procedure for disposable flat-plate (cellulosic) dialyzers is similar to that used for hollow-fiber dialyzers, but includes use of a cleaning agent, warm 1% bleach for a maximum of 5 min. Flat-plate dialyzers are used, on the average, four times.

Rogers et al. [20] of the Hattiesburg Clinic in Mississippi have described their procedure for reusing hollow-fiber dialyzers, which employs hydrogen peroxide as a cleaning agent:

1. Blood is returned to the patient with 200 ml of heparinized saline.
2. The dialyzer is flushed with water and then with 3% hydrogen peroxide. This is repeated if the dialyzer is not clean.
3. After volume testing (minimum 90% of original), the dialyzer is filled with water and then 10% formalin (4% HCHO).
4. To prepare for use, the dialyzer is first rinsed with 500 ml of saline with dialysate flowing through the dialysate compartment. The saline, arterial, and venous lines are connected by a three-way valve and flow is recirculated as saline is infused into the circuit while dialyzing against a negative pressure (500 mmHg) for 15 min.

The dialyzers were capable of being reused an average of 4–6 times in two groups of patients.

The reuse procedure employed by the Regional Kidney Disease Program in Minneapolis [7] also employs hydrogen peroxide (H_2O_2) as a cleaning agent:

1. Rinse dialyzers with a minimum of 2 liters of water.
2. Clean with 0.6% H_2O_2.
3. Perform volume and pressure test.
4. Fill blood compartment with 500 ml of 4% HCHO.
5. Rinse out until no HCHO detected by Hantzsch reaction (< 1 ppm).

In their study, dialyzers were reused three times.

The manual reprocessing method employed by Kaye et al. [21] at the Montreal General Hospital includes the use of bleach:

1. Rinse blood compartment until clear (10–40 min) and then rinse the dialysate compartment with H_2O at 70 mmHg.
2. Apply reverse ultrafiltration (50 mmHg on dialysate side).
3. Flush blood compartment 2–3 min and then fill with 1.0% sodium hypochlorite (NaOCl) for 1 min.
4. Rinse 5 min and then fill with 4.0% HCHO.
5. Prepare for use with a 30-min flush of the dialysate compartment and then rinse the blood compartment with 500 ml saline.

When an automated device was used which employed 4.3% NaOCl, Kaye et al. [21] were able to obtain, on the average, 16 reuses of the Gambro 120M dialyzer. They reported no change in clearance of urea, creatinine, and phosphate in up to 30 uses.

Bourke et al. [22] and Matthew et al. [23] at the Queen Elizabeth Hospital in Australia describe their procedure as follows:

1. Flush dialyzers with RO water (10 psi) until HEMASTIC® reaction is negative.
2. Store dialyzer in 3% HCHO.
3. Flush with saline until CLINITEST® negative.

FBVs were not routinely measured. Heparin dosage was individually tailored and was maintained at a constant dosage, the mean dose per treatment being 4500 untis. With this procedure, 12 uses of the Asahi AM10 dialyzer were possible with no compromise in performance.

The procedure used by Heonich et al. [24] at the Royal Victoria Infirmary in Newcastle upon Tyne is:

1. Begin reprocessing immediately after disconnecting patient.

2. Rinse dialyzer with RO-treated water, periodically clamping the dialysate outflow (to produce momentary reverse ultrafiltration into the blood compartment). Continue until rinse from blood compartment is clear (8−10 min).
3. Fill dialyzer with 2% HCHO.
4. To prepare for use, rinse dialysate compartment for 1 h with tap H_2O. Prior to connecting the patient, rinse blood compartment with sterile 0.9% saline. After 900 ml, test with Schiff Reagent.

Dialyzers were discarded if FBV decreased more than 10% or if dialyzers were discolored, damaged, or reprocessed improperly. They found that 72% of dialyzers were reused twice and 36% five times with this procedure. (See chapter 8 for more details.)

The following procedure is employed by the National Nephrology Foundation and is based on our earlier studies [4]:

1. Deliver dialyzer filled with heparinized saline to storage area within 10 min of disconnection from patient.
2. Flush blood side with RO water for 5 min (20 psi, 3−4 liters/min, A− to V− direction, A− side down).
3. Cleanse blood side by repeating four times over a 1-h period a cycle of reverse ultrafiltration and flushing with RO water: (a) the dialysate side is first filled with RO water (the direction of fill alternates with each cycle), air pockets and bubbles are removed, and then the outflow line is clamped for 15 min; (b) the dialysate flow is released and the blood compartment is rinsed for 2 min with RO water (20 psi, 3−4 liters/min), during which time the outflow is clamped briefly three times.
4. The dialyzer is volume tested. It is discarded if FBV is less than 80% of original or if it contains many clotted fibers.
5. The dialyzer is filled with 2% HCHO.
6. To prepare for use, HCHO is removed under a fume hood in the storage area by flushing the dialysate compartment with RO water (minimum flow 100 ml/min for 10 min). In the treatment area, lines are connected and the dialysate side is flushed for at least 10 min with 500 ml/min dialysate (A− to V− direction, V− side down) (negative pressure set to 0).
7. The blood side is flushed with 500 ml heparinized saline (2000 IU/liter; flow rate 125 ml/min) and then the venous side is clamped while flow continues through the dialysate side for at least 10 min more (negative pressure still 0).
8. The dialyzer is inverted and the blood side is flushed with an additional 500 ml saline.
9. The dialyzer is CLINITEST®-ed and pressure tested before use.

This method has been used with modifications on two high-flux type cellulosic hemodialyzers, the Cordis Dow Duo-flux and the Travenol CA-170. It is our experience that negative pressure must be carefully controlled during reverse ultrafiltration or the fibers tend to collapse. Typically three reuses can be obtained, while for conventional cellulose membranes a target of 12 uses is employed.

Polyacrylonitrile (PAN) membranes

Devices in current use that employ the PAN membrane include the Rhone-Poulenc AN-69 hemofilter, the Asahi PAN 150, and Hospal 3000 S.

Hemofiltration tends to produce a protein cake on the membrane, especially in the postdilution mode, which may be difficult to remove with standard reprocessing techniques.

Reprocessing of PAN devices has been reported by Vercellone et al. [25], Van Holder [26], Aljama et al. [27], and Andreucci et al. [28].

Andreucci et al. [28] reused the RP 610 five times with AMUCHINA® (hypochlorous acid in 18% NaCl) as disinfectant. Their procedure is as follows:

1. The hemofilter is washed with 500 ml of saline containing 5000 IU heparin.
2. The dialyzer is cleaned with 5 liters of 5% AMUCHINA® over a 20− to 40−min period, inverting several times and constricting the blood-side flow intermittently. Reverse ultrafiltration is employed to clean the blood compartment.
3. The dialyzer is filled with 300 ml of 5% AMUCHINA® and stored at 4°C for 48−72 h until next use.
4. For reuse the dialyzer is flushed with 1 liter of saline.

Both in vivo and in vitro clearances and hydraulic permeability were measured, and were maintained through five reuses of the RP 610 hemofilter.

Polysulphone (PS) membranes

Examples of devices using this material include the Amicon A20 diafilter and the Fresenius F60 filter [29]. Zbinder and Binswanger [30] have described reuse of the Fresenius F60 membrane. They used the Renatron reprocessing device, cleaning the membranes with 3% peracetic acid (RENALIN®), and then storing in 2% HCHO. The dialyzer was flushed with 3 liters saline before use. The F60 was discarded if priming volume decreased more than 12% of the initial value. The number of reuses varied from a few to 19. Clearances were maintained and no side effects were evident.

Polymethylmethacrylate (PMMA) membranes

We are not aware of published methods for reprocessing devices made with this material.

Polypropylene (PP) membranes

No reprocessing methods are known to us for devices made with this material.

Polycarbonate membranes

Hemmeloff et al. 1985 [31] recently described the performance of the Gambro GAMBRANE® polycarbonate flat-sheet hemodialyzer, but reprocessing methods have not yet been reported.

RATIONALE FOR PROCEDURES

Prerinse procedures

Mean usage of hemodialyzers may be related to the specifics of anticoagulation of both the patient and the saline used to return blood to the patient. Unfortunately, there have been very few reports directed toward optimizing heparin usage for reprocessing of hemodialyzers. How much time should elapse after giving the patient heparin before connecting the patient to the dialyzer? Is there any advantage to continuous heparin infusion? It is our experience that dialyzers of certain patients do not reprocess as well as those of other patients. Viljoen et al. [32] regard heparin dosage as not being critical, and others have commented [33, 34] that dialyzers of certain patients tend to clot no matter how much heparin is given. On the other hand, there are those who consider heparin quite important and who tailor heparin dosage to each patient [22]. It is probably true that the heparin schedule is not critical for obtaining a few satisfactory reuses, but we do not know how important it is for extending mean usage far beyond that.

It is generally regarded that during the saline (heparinized saline) rinse-back of blood to the patient, air should not be allowed to enter the dialyzer. This step is not easy to control and is probably subject to error.

Another early step in reprocessing that is subject to variability is the time interval between disconnection of the patient and the initiation of the rinsing procedure, and the temperature of the dialyzer during this time interval. Some consider that this interval should be kept to the very minimum [6, 24], while others find it possible to set aside or refrigerate the dialyzer. Billiouw et al. [35], for example, find it possible to rinse-back the dialyzer with 500 ml of heparinized saline (5000 IU/liter) and store the dialyzer at 4°C until it is convenient to begin reprocessing. The AAMI draft of recommended practice [3] on reuse states a consensus that delays longer than 6 h may be acceptable if physiological solution is used to return blood to the patient and the dialyzer is refrigerated. Ferreira et al. [36], on the other hand, consider it important to avoid exposing the dialyzer to cool temperatures prior to rinsing.

Dechelette et al. [37] reused the Kuraray SA plasmafilter (a polyvinyl acetate membrane) up to 16 times and recommended immediate rinse after use, but saw no urgency to the rest of the procedure.

Rinsing

The objective of rinsing the dialyzer after use is to remove as much blood as possible without at the same time producing fibrin deposits in the fibers. It seems preferable that this be done with heparinized saline of the same temperature as the dialyzer immediately after disconnecting the patient. In practice, water is used instead of saline, except for the initial rinse-back of blood to the patient, and its temperature is often much less than that of the dialyzer. As noted above, some have refrigerated the dialyzer prior to rinse, so this aspect of the reuse procedure may not be critical.

Extensive bidirectional rinsing with application of reverse ultrafiltration has been used in many facilities to flush residual blood from the dialyzer fibers. This procedure is often used in lieu of a separate cleaning step, at least in manual procedures. This seems satisfactory for reusing dialyzers 6−10 times without significant degradation of performance, but whether it suffices for much larger numbers of reuses is not documented.

Previously Deane and Bemis [4] compared a simple rinse procedure with a complex one, and found no difference in clearances and ultrafiltration of dialyzers after one use. More recently, Meftahi et al. [38] used another approach, high-pressure liquid chromatographic analysis of rinse eluates, to evaluate rinsing procedures; 62 CUPROPHAN® dialyzers from seven manufacturers were tested. They report that rinsing is favored by elevated temperature (37°C) and a static mode of rinse.

The rinsing phase of the reuse procedure deserves further study because of indications that intradialytic symptoms are related to residues from the manufacturing process [14, 38]. Recently evidence has been presented implicating residues of ETO sterilization that bind to the polyurethane potting compound in dialyzers in hypersensitivity reactions.

Although rinsing and cleaning solutions are rarely, if ever, degassed for reuse, there is general agreement among practitioners that as much air should be removed as is practical from the dialyzer during rinsing and succeeding steps. Viljoen et al. [32] reported that filling the dialyzer with formaldehyde after a negative pressure had been applied to degas the blood compartment produced fewer clotted fibers and increased performance and reuse statistics markedly. For successful reuse, Gotch [34] considers important the degassing of the blood compartment prior to filling with sterilant or a cleaning agent.

Water for reprocessing of dialyzers is used not only for rinsing blood and dialysate compartments, but also for preparation and rinse out of any blood compartment cleaning solutions that might be employed and for preparing disinfectant and dialysate solutions. Thus, there is appropriate concern for the levels of organics, inorganics, bacteria, and endotoxins that may be present in this water. According to the AAMI recommended practice [3], water used for reprocessing of hemodialyzers should be analyzed periodically to insure compatibility with acceptable dialysis techniques. Some states specifically require that the water meet the AAMI standard (see chapter 12).

Because some measurements of biocompatibility, and outcome of reuse, may be influenced by endotoxin levels in the dialyzer or dialysis solutions, it is worth emphasizing that endotoxin levels should be documented in studies of reprocessing techniques. Rarely has this been done in published reports. It is encouraging that one manufactuer of analysis kits reports that more than 50 dialysis units regularly test their dialysis water for endotoxin levels (Gould, Associates of Cape Cod, Inc., personal communication).

Cleaning

Should the reuse procedure be designed to restore the hemodialyzer to its original condition, or should one try to obtain a dialyzer that may be superior to a new one? This question regarding the real intent of a reprocessing procedure is brought into focus by the issue of whether or not sodium hypochlorite should be used, and if so, at what concentration. If a reprocessing procedure is intended to restore the dialyzer membrane to its original condition, then bleach may be useful. On the other hand, if increased biocompatibility is desired, then bleach should probably be eliminated or be used at very low concentrations for a short time interval.

There are numerous reports showing that the leukopenia that occurs 10–15 minutes into hemodialysis with cellulosic membranes decreases with repeated use of the dialyzer, provided that bleach is not used to clean the dialyzer [9, 24, 41–43]. Gagnon and Kaye [42] observed that neutropenia reappears when the concentration of bleach increases from 1% to 4.3%, the latter concentration being used in some automated devices. Dorson et al. [44] found that as little as 0.25% NaOCl decreased the burst strength of CUPROPHAN® membranes. Rancourt et al. [43] reported that neutropenia and intradialytic symptoms analogous to those of first use appear when 0.6% NaOCl is used to clean cellulose acetate and saponified cellulose ester membranes. The dialyzers did not show any increase in rupture or leak rate when used 10–15 times. Deane and Bemis [4] earlier showed that 5.25% bleach, while an effective cleanser of dialyzers, reacts with these membranes exothermically, causing ultrafiltration and clearances to be enhanced.

Of the various membrane materials in use, CUPROPHAN® and cellulose acetate react with NaOCl while PAN membranes are not affected under similar conditions of exposure [45].

Hydrogen peroxide is another chemical employed as a cleaning agent of dialyzers. We previously found it to be rather ineffective [4], but its use continues, especially in automated devices. RENALIN®, consisting of peracetic acid and hydrogen peroxide, is said to be a cleaning agent as well as a disinfectant [47], but this may be from the hydrogen peroxide that is present. The latter reacts with the heme group of hemoglobin, causing the red color to disappear without actually removing protein from the filter, unlike treatment with NaOCl. The visual cleanliness of peroxide-cleaned (or peracetic-acid-cleaned) dialyzers may thus be deceiving.

Dialyzer assessment

Hollow-fiber dialyzers have largely replaced flat-plate and coil-type dialyzers because of the ease with which function can be measured in these devices. The priming volume (total cell volume, TCV; or fiber bundle volume, FBV) is taken to be directly proportional to the number of functional fibers (see chapter 3). This volume can be measured readily by manual or automated methods. According to Gotch [15], clearances of clinically important small molecules (mol. wt. 60−160) decrease 4% to 11% when the decrease in total cell volume is limited to 20%.

Dorson [10] and Dorson et al. [44], while not ruling out the usefulness of TCV, consider that ultrafiltration rate (UFR) provides a more sensitive measure of residual dialyzer function, especially for characterizing mass transport of larger molecular weight species. They consider that TCV is useful to follow clotting of fibers, and UFR is useful to follow protein deposition in the fiber. (See discussions in chapters 3 and 12.)

Ultrafiltration measurements can be automated, and five of the six reprocessing devices we tested [8] incorporated UFR into the protocol for dialyzer assessment.

There have been recommendations [11] that pressure testing be performed on all reprocessed dialyzers to eliminate the possibility of leaking membranes. The occurrence of leaking dialyzers may be lower for reprocessed dialyzers than for new dialyzers [3], however, because defective dialyzers are initially selected out. On the other hand, use of a strong cleaning agent (NaOCl, for example) could degrade the membrane, especially with repeated use, and pressure testing is then recommended.

The performance of reprocessed high-flux dialyzers must be adequately documented, particularly as regards leak rate, because reverse ultrafiltration over part of the membranes is said to occur [48], making contamination from the dialysate side possible.

Methodological questions of dialyzer assessment aside, there is the issue of whether or not reprocessed dialyzers transport larger molecules to a lesser extent than new dialyzers and, if so, what the long-term consequences might be. This could have an impact on future methods for assessment of dialyzer function.

Sterilization (disinfection)

The microbiologic organisms of greatest concern in the dialysis setting include water-adapted gram-negative bacteria and nontuberculous mycobacteria [16, 47, 49, 50]. The latter are reported to be present in untreated water in 83% of the centers surveyed by the CDC [2]. Bacterial spores are not considered to be a problem and sporicidal agents are believed not to be required. (See chapter 4 for more detail.)

The most common microbiologic hazard associated with reprocessing of dialyzers is not bacteremia, however, but endotoxemia [1, 47, 49] originating from gram-negative organisms present in standing, facility water or from unpurified system water. The AAMI Recommended Practice [3] and the NKF Revised Standards [11] state that water used to prepare disinfectant solutions should contain less than 1 ng/ml endotoxin (limulus amoebocyte lysate [LAL] reactive material) and should be tested at least monthly. A possible rationale for the use of water, essentially free_ of endotoxin, for dilution of formaldehyde is that formaldehyde may chemically bind endotoxin to the membrane or other surface within the blood compartment. Thus the requirement for dilution water to have less than 1 ng/ml of endotoxin is critically important. The same rationale may apply to other aldehyde based sterilant/disinfectants.

Most hemodialysis facilities in the United States that reprocess dialyzers use formaldehyde as disinfectant [1], 38% using 2% HCHO according to the 1983 CDC survey [2] and 23% using 4% HCHO. Although infections from nontuberculous mycobacteria are not common in these patients, and no endotoxin is produced by their presence, 4% HCHO is now recommended in the AAMI Recommended Practice [3] and the NKF Standards [11] to prevent growth of these organisms. However, rinsing out the HCHO to the recommended level of 5 µg/ml (5 ppm) or less, recommended in the AAMI draft practice [3], becomes substantially more time consuming and expensive when 4% HCHO is employed [15].

Despite the long record of success of formaldehyde as an effective disinfecting agent for reprocessing dialyzers, the search continues for better alternatives. The chemicals being most actively investigated include gluteraldehyde-based formulations (CIDEX® and SPORICIDIN®), peroxyacetic acid solutions (RENALIN®), and active chlorine compounds (WAREXIN®, RENNEW-D®, and AMUCHINA®) (see table 2—1). The higher molecular weight sterilants might be effective at lower concentrations, but their interaction with, and diffusion from, the components of the dialyzer determine the ease with which these materials can be removed prior to reuse.

CIDEX® (CIDEX-HD, Surgikos) is an alkaline solution of glutaraldehyde (table 2—1) that, according to the manufacturer, is fungicidal, virucidal, and sporicidal, and is compatible with cellulosic dialyzer membranes. Petersen et al. [51] reported that it is effective against the atypical water mycobacteria and other organisms that might contaminate hemodialysis systems. It does not contain a phenolic substance, as does SPORICIDIN® (table 2—1), and washes out from cellulosic dialyzers more easily than does formaldehyde, according to impressions gained in the clinical trials conducted for the manufacturer.

Since a liquid disinfectant introduced into a dialyzer may not be able to

Table 2-1. Chemicals being most actively investigated as a disinfecting agent for reprocessing dialyzers.

Disinfectant	Source	Active ingredient	Properties
Formaldehyde	—	2% 4%	Low-level disinfectant High-level disinfectant
CIDEX®-HD	Surgikos, Inc. Arlington, TX	0.8% alkaline glutaraldehyde	Fungicidal, virucidal, sporicidal; nonmutagenic
SPORICIDIN®	Sporicidin, Inc. Washington, DC	0.15% glutaraldehyde plus 0.5% sodium phenate	Sporicidal, virucidal
RENALIN®	Renal Systems, Inc. Minneapolis, MN	0.5% peracetic acid (peracetic acid, hydrogen peroxide and acetic acid)	Fungicidal, virucidal, sporicidal
WAREXIN®	Mediflex International, Inc. West Caldwell, NJ	Monoxychlorosene; tetra decylbenzenesulfonate— hypochlorous acid complex, 0.125% or 0.250%	Sporicidal
REN-NEW-D® (ALCIDE)	Alcide Corp. Westport, CT	Chlorine dioxide	Fungicidal, virucidal, sporicidal; nonmutagenic
AMUCHINA®	Amuchina. S.p.A. Genoa, Italy	Trace hypochlorous acid in 18% NaCl: 11 ppm active chlorine	Fungicidal virucidal, sporicidal; nontoxic

diffuse to all surface areas of the device, an important consideration when choosing an alternative disinfectant is the activity of the vapor toward the various organisms of interest. The CIDEX® vapor is more effective than that of 4% formaldehyde toward the atypical water mycobacteria, according to Wendt et al. [52] of Surgikos. In a summary of two studies sponsored by Surgikos, Wendt et al. [52] report no adverse effects of CIDEX-HD® on cellulosic membranes, as measured by clearances, particles shedding, and membrane strength. Additionally no adverse effects on patients treated with CIDEX-HD® reprocessed dialyzers were noted.

We have attempted to test the efficacy of various alternative sterilants in standard cellulosic dialyzers by inoculating the dialyzer with different water-adapted bacteria. Although we were not able to start with colony counts of 10^6/ml for this study, to obtain 6-log kills, we were able to show that CIDEX® and 4% formaldehyde required only 1 h to inactivate the organisms. In contrast, 2% formaldehyde required 24 h, while REN-NEW-D® and WAREXIN® (see table 2−1) required only 20 min.

SPORICIDIN® (Table 2−1) contains both glutaraldehyde and sodium phenate as active ingredients. Hakim has reported on the use of SPORICIDIN® in automated reprocessing of hemodialyzers [54]. Gotch [15] measured the rinse-out kinetics of sodium phenate and calculated that removing SPORICIDIN® would be somewhat more difficult than removing 4% HCHO from cellulosic dialyzers.

Per(oxy)acetic acid is available commercially as RENALIN® (table 2−1), and consists of an equilibrium mixture of peracetic acid, acetic acid, and hydrogen peroxide. It is virucidal, fungicidal, and sporicidal, killing organisms by oxidation of enzymes. De Palma [55] reprocessed dialyzers up to 30 times when storing with 500−1000 ppm RENALIN®, obtaining a mean usage of 17 with this disinfectant. Use of RENALIN® for disinfecting hemodialyzers is reported to give fewer intradialytic symptoms as compared with disinfection with HCHO [9, 47]. Endotoxin present in CUPROPHAN® dialyzers has been shown to decrease upon repeated reprocessing with RENALIN® [56], as it does with formaldehyde reprocessing [47, 57].

Berkseth et al. [46] and Bauer et al. [58] reprocessed CUPROPHAN® dialyzers using the RENATRON®, which employs RENALIN® both as a cleaning agent and as a disinfectant. Berkseth et al. stored their dialyzers at 4°C until next use because of the decomposition of peracetic acid in the presence of organics. They noted that RENALIN® made their CUPROPHAN® dialyzers appear cleaner, presumably from the effect of H_2O_2 on the heme group of hemoglobin.

The 1984 survey of dialysis facilities [1] did not demonstrate a clear advantage of peracetic acid as a cleaning agent. Mean usage was somewhat higher when peracetic acid was used (ten reuses vs eight for HCHO alone), but the difference was not statistically significant, as the mean number of reuses ranged from one to 19 in facilities using this technique, far greater than for any other procedure. No procedure showed a clear advantage over any other, however, in terms of increasing mean usage of dialyzers.

WAREXIN® is a nontoxic sporicidal agent. It contains buffered hypochlorous acid, which oxidizes proteinaceous material in the dialyzer. It is not stable at room temperature and solutions must be used within 72 h after preparation from a dry powder. Dialyzers stored in WAREXIN® are normally kept at 4°C. The vapor retains its effectiveness against bacteria. WAREXIN® can be measured by the potassium iodide titration method.

REN-NEW-D® is a compound that produces chlorine dioxide "on demand" upon interaction with organic material. It is not toxic, mutagenic, or teratogenic in standard toxicology tests, and it does not irritate or stain the skin.

Wineman et al. 1985 [53] have investigated possible effects of REN-NEW-D (ALCIDE®) on CUPROPHAN®, cellulose acetate, and saponified cellulose acetate membranes in an in vitro study. Usage was simulated by recirculating anticoagulated blood through the dialyzers. Clearances of creatinine, urea, and B_{12} remained within 3%−12% of initial values, while FBV decreased less than 10% after up to 20 simulated uses. Ultrafiltration increased on the average 20%, with some diminution in burts strength of the dialyzers.

Two clinical studies of ALCIDE® are in progress. Kaye (personal communication) finds that ALCIDE® is as effective as HCHO for repeated use of dialyzers. The manufacturer's claim that ALCIDE® is a cleaning agent is substantiated by the finding that the FBV of rejected dialyzers can be increased by treatment with ALCIDE®, analogous to our findings with sodium hypochlorite [4]. Kaye considers that ALCIDE® is a good cleaning agent, though not as strong as bleach.

Swenson (personal communication) reports being able to obtain 20 reuses with CUPROPHAN® dialyzers stored in ALCIDE®, with a mean of about 15 reuses. He finds ALCIDE® to be as effective as formaldehyde when NaOCl is used as a cleaning agent.

The disinfectant AMUCHINA® is a stable solution of hypochlorous acid in 18% NaOCl, produced by Amuchina S.p.A. in Genoa, Italy (table 2-1). According to information supplied by the manufacturer, it is fungicidal, virucidal, and sporicidal [59, 60] and nontoxic even when ingested. Lamperi et al. [61] used AMUCHINA® with hemodialyzers and reported that, after one reuse, dialyzers stored in AMUCHINA® were cleaner, by visual and electron-microscopic examination, than dialyzers stored in formaldehyde. Andreucci et al. [28] used the Rhone Poulene RP 610 for postdilution hemofiltration, and reported reprocessing the devices up to five times without significantly altering the characteristics of the membranes.

Preparation for next use

Preparing a dialyzer for use consists of flushing out the disinfectant to reduce the residual sterilant concentration to below maximum recommended levels. For HCHO this level is taken as 5 ppm [3], although levels of 10 ppm and 1 ppm also have been recommended (see chapters 3 and 9). Since the tests to document the levels are not always easy to perform in a clinical setting, random testing is sometimes employed. Other facilities test all dialyzers with the less sensitive, but more convenient, CLINITEST® tablet after having verified by appropriately sensitive tests that the recommended standard of performance can be met when the rinse-out procedure is performed properly.

It should be kept in mind that hypersensitivity to residues from the manufacturing process [14, 38, 39, 42] may occur, as well as endotoxemia from gram-negative organisms present at one time in the water used to reprocess or manufacture the dialyzer [4, 47, 49, 56, 57], and these factors also have to be monitored on a regular basis. There is increasing evidence that hypersensitivity reactions in some patients are from residues of ethylene oxide sterilization [39, 40, 62]. The LAL-reactive material that may occur in high concentrations in CUPROPHAN® dialyzers [63], and that is leached out with each use [4, 47, 57, 58], may not always be pyrogenic [62, 64, 65]. Yamagami et al. [64] reported that LAL-reactive material, which was absent from dialyzers having PMMA membranes, had a beta-glucone-like structure, unlike that of the endotoxin.

Dorson [10] recently showed that hundreds of hours of rinsing are required to reduce the LAL-reactive material occurring in CUPROPHAN® membranes below detection levels of $0.008-0.013$ ng/ml. Interestingly, two-thirds of patients still exhibited dialysis-induced neutropenia when treated with these exhaustively rinsed dialyzers. Although the recommended maximum level of LAL-reaction material is 1 ng/ml [3] in water used to dilute formaldehyde, it should be noted that Pitt et al. [66] report that 0.3 ng/ml *Escherichia coli* endotoxin still produces substantial generation of factor C3a.

Formaldehyde does not rinse out of cellulosic dialyzers easily because it binds to the polyurethane potting compound in the headers [17]. Gotch and Keen recommend that rinsing be done at 37°C to decrease residual levels of HCHO to appropriate amounts. The "initial burst" phenomenon, which can be demonstrated by stopping flow from a rinsed dialyzer and later releasing it, is well known [4]. Lewis et al. [67] and Kaye et al. [68] report milligram quantities of HCHO entering the patient after the concentration of HCHO in the eluate was reduced below $1-2$ µg/ml. The latter workers recently investigated either different rinse out protocols with 2.7% and 4% HCHO as disinfectants and report being able to obtain acceptable concentrations (< 0.5 µg/ml) 95% of the time after a 45-min rinse-out procedure, with dialyzers reused up to 21 times. A factor that has not been documented in most descriptions of reprocessing is the total amount of HCHO that can be expected to enter the patient following a standard rinse-out procedure. This information is needed to develop a standard of practice.

According to preliminary data of the manufacturers, rinsing out CIDEX® from cellulosic dialyzers is easier than rinsing out HCHO, indicating that glutaraldehyde does not bind as tightly to the membrane−polyurethane margins. A residual test kit is available from the manufacturer that permits measurement to 1 ppm in 1 min. FDC blue dye no. 1 can be used to indicate both the presence of CIDEX® in the dialyzer and, roughly, its removal following rinse out.

Hakim [54] has reported the kinetics of rinse out of glutaraldehyde and sodium phenate from reprocessed dialyzers. He found that glutaraldehyde rinses out faster than formaldehyde, but the phenate component of SPORICIDIN® is harder to remove, as shown earlier by Gotch [15].

Particulates

There have been few studies documenting levels of particulates in the effluent from dialyzers prepared for use. Deane and Bemis [4] measured particulates eluting from new and multiply used CUPROPHAN® dialyzers, and found no significant difference. Keshaviah et al. [5, 69] also have reported particulate levels.

CONCLUSIONS

Those procedural steps that seem to be the most important for improving the reprocessing of hemodialyzers and hemofilters are the following:

1. Prompt reprocessing after use.
2. Thorough removal of air bubbles from the blood compartment during rinsing, possibly to include degassing the blood compartment prior to filling the blood compartment with sterilant.
3. Application of reverse ultrafiltration to dislodge materials in the blood compartment. Cleaning by reverse ultrafiltration becomes more difficult with newer membranes having high ultrafiltration rates and noncompliant fibers.
4. Rinsing procedures that remove various residues from the manufacturing and sterilization process known to be present in dialyzers rinsed by standard procedures.
5. Use of endotoxin-free water to prepare disinfectant solutions.
6. Rinse-out procedures that document total residual disinfectant (bioburden) remaining in the dialyzer after preparation for next use.

The elements of reprocessing that require further study, in addition to the above, include the following:

1. Dose and schedule of heparin administration (or other anticoagulant) for increasing number of reuses.
2. Long-term effects, if any, of the newer sterilants.
3. The role of specific protein deposition onto the dialyzer membrane in observations of enhanced biocompatibility with reuse. This needs to be disinguished from the beneficial effects resulting from removal of manufacturing residues and endotoxins during reprocessing.

Quality control of the reprocessing procedure has not been mentioned, not because we think it is unimportant, but because it is discussed elsewhere in this volume. For many dialysis facilities, including our own, it is probably true that careful attention to quality control alone will improve reuse statistics and contribute to improved patient care.

REFERENCES

1. Deane N: A survey of dialyzer reuse practice in the United States—1984. AAMI Technical Assessment Report 10—85. Hemodialyzer reuse: issues and solutions. Association for the Advancement of Medical Instrumentation, Arlington VA, 1985, pp 1—5.
2. Bland LA, Alter MJ, Favero MS, Carson LA, Cusick LB: Hemodialyzer reuse: practices in the United States and implication for infection control [abstr]. Am Soc Artif Intern Organs 14:40, 1985.
3. Association for the Advancement of Medical Instrumentation: AAMI recommended practice for reuse of hemodialyzers (draft). Association for the Advancement of Medical Instrumentation, Arlington VA, 1984.
4. Deane N, Bemis J: Multiple use of hemodialyzers: final report to the National Institutes of Arthritis, Diabetes and Digestive and Kidney Disease. Contract NO1-AM-9-2214, June 1981, pp 53—64.
5. Keshaviah PD, Luehmann D, Shapiro F, Comty C: Investigation of the risks and hazards associated with hemodialysis systems. Technical Report, contract 223-78-5046. US Department of Health and Human Services, Public Health Service/Food and Drug Administration/Bureau of Medical Devices, Silver Springs MD, June 1980.
6. Sadler JH (ed): National workshop on reuse of consumables in hemodialysis. Kidney Disease Coalition, Washington DC, 1983.
7. Stroncek DF, Keshaviah P, Craddock PR, Hammerschmidt DE: Effect of dialyzer reuse on complement activation and neutropenia in hemodialysis. J Lab Clin Med 104:304—311, 1984.
8. Deane N, Wineman RJ: Comparative evaluation of automated devices for reprocessing hemodialyzers: intradialytic patient response. Trans Am Soc Artif Intern Organs 30:498—501, 1984.
9. Jayashankar JE, Karfonta S, Venkatachalam K, Deegan MJ: Effect of method of dialyzer reprocessing on complement activation, leucopenia, and symptoms during hemodialysis: a randomized controlled study [abstr]. Am Soc Artif Intern Organs 14:57, 1985.
10. Dorson WJ: Biocompatibility, leachables and membrane structure. Trans Am Soc Artif Intern Organs 30:715—717, 1984.
11. National Kidney Foundation: Revised standards for reuse of hemodialyzers. Am J Kidney Dis 3:466—468, 1984.
12. Ogden DA: New dialyzer syndrome. N Engl J Med 302:1262—1263, 1980.
13. Klinkmann H, Ivanovich P: Dialysis: advantages and disadvantages of current dialysis techniques. In: Nephrology, vol 2: 9th International congress of nephrology. Springer-Verlag, New York, 1984, pp 1528—1552.
14. Kuentz F, Foret M, Hachache T, Christollet M, Milongo R, Meftachi H, Dechelette E, Cordonnier D: Hypersensitivity reactions during hemodialysis in France [abstr]. Eur Dial Transplant Assoc, 1985, p 118.
15. Gotch FA: Dialyzer transport properties and sterilant elution. In: Deane N, Wineman RJ (eds) Seminar on reuse of hemodialyzers: automated and manual methods. National Nephrology Foundation, New York, 1984, p 10.
16. Band JD, Wood JI, Fraser DW, Petersen NJ, et al.: Peritonitis caused by a mycobacterium chelonei-like organism associated with chronic peritoneal dialysis. J Infect Dis 145:9—17, 1982.
17. Gotch F, Keen M: Formaldehyde kinetics in reused dialyzers. Trans Am Soc Artif Intern Organs 29:396—401, 1983.
18. Sakai K, Mimura R, Takesawa S, Ozawa K: Pore diameter of small tubular membranes currently used in hemodialysis [abstr]. Am Soc Artif Intern Organs 14:36, 1985.
19. Blagg CR: Home dialysis and dialyzer reuse in Seattle. In: Sadler J (ed) Proceedings of the

national workshop on the reuse of consumables in hemodialysis. Kidney Disease Coalition, Washington DC, 1983, pp 40–47.

20. Rogers PW, Gersh HA, Sims CE, Ellis J: Experience with dialyzer reuse in a community hemodialysis unit. In: Sadler J (ed) Proceedings of the national Workshop on the reuse of consumables in hemodialysis. Kidney Disease Coalition, Washington DC, 1983, pp 54–61.

21. Kaye M, Gagnon R, Mulhearn B, Spergel D: Prolonged dialyzer reuse. Trans Am Soc Artif Intern Organs 30:491–493, 1984.

22. Bourke MA, Matthew TH, Fazzalari RA, Thislwell G, Disney APS: Multiple use of dialyzers: six uses is the optimum. Med J Aust 140:10–12, 1984.

23. Matthew TH, Fazzalari RA, Disney APS, MacIntyre DB: Multiple use of dialyzers: an Australian view. Nephron 27:222–225, 1981.

24. Heonich NA, Johnson SR, Buckley P, Harden J, Ward MK, Kerr DN: Haemodialyser reuse: impact on function and biocompatibility. Int J Artif Organs 6:261–266, 1983.

25. Vercellone A, et al.: Reuse of dialyzers: PAN reuse. Dial Transplant 7:350, 1978.

26. Van Holder R: Two years experience with automated reprocessing of hemofilters and hemodialyzers. Paper presented at the International Workshop on Hemodialyzer Reprocessing, 21 September 1984, Bad Homburg, FRG. (to be published).

27. Aljama P, Bird PA, Ward MK, Feest TG, Walker W, Tanboga H, Sussman M, Kerr DN: Hemodialysis-induced leukopenia and activation of complement: effects of different membranes. Proc Eur Dial Transplant Assoc 15:144–153, 1978.

28. Andreucci VE, Calderano V, Merroli B, et al.: Concentration polarization phenomenon in new and re-used RP 610 hemofilters during post dilutional hemofiltration. Int J Artif Organs 3:147–157, 1980.

29. Schneider H, Streicher E: Mass transfer characterization of a new polysulfone membrane. Artif Organs 9:180–183, 1985.

30. Zbinden M, Binswanger U: Reuse of polysulfone capillary filters [abstr]. Eur Dial Transplant Assoc, 1985, p 142.

31. Hemmeloff KE, Riede G, Konstantin P, Gohl H: The performance and compatibility of a new copolymeric membrane—Gambrane—for hemodialysis [abstr]. Eur Dial Transplant Assoc 1985, p 114.

32. Viljoen M, Gold CH, Burgess HR: The importance of degassing the hollow fiber artificial kidney (HFAK) for multiple reuse. Nephron 28:46–49, 1981.

33. Soberman R: National workshop on reuse of consumables in hemodialysis. Kidney Disease Coalition, Washington DC, 1983, p 65.

34. Gotch F: Reprocessing technology for dialyzers using manual and automated techniques. Paper presented at the International Workshop on Hemodialyzer Reprocessing, 21 September 1984, Bad Homburg, FRG (to be published).

35. Billiouw JM, Van Holder R, Piron M, Veirman R, Ringoir S: Automated reuse of capillary hemodialyzers. Int J Artif Organs 8:83–88, 1985.

36. Ferreira C, Martins R, Oliveira L, Paz R, Pratas J: Factors which interfere in the reprocessing of dialyzers in an automatic reuse programme [abstr]. Eur Dial Transplant Assoc, 1985, p 111.

37. Dechelette E, Lambert CL, Bessoud Y, Kuentz F, Jurkovitz CL: Argument for the reuse of plasmafilter [abstr]. Eur Dial Transplant Assoc, 1985, p 144.

38. Meftahi H, et al.: HPLC study of cuprophan hollow-fiber dialysers extracts: determination of an optimal rinsing procedure [abstr]. Eur Dial Transplant Assoc, 1985, p 124.

39. Henne W, Schulze H, Pelger M, Tretzel J, Von Sengbusch G: Hollow-fiber dialyzers and their pyrogenicity testing by limulus amoebocyte lysate. Artif Organs 8:299–305, 1984.

40. Lee FF, Leonard EE: Urethanes as ethylene oxide reservoirs in hollow fibre dialysers [abstr]. Eur Dial Transplant Assoc, 1985, p 119.

41. Kant KS, Pollack VE, Chathey M, Goetz D, Berlin R, et al.: Multiple use of dialyzers: safety and efficacy. Kidney Int 19:728–738, 1981.

42. Gagnon RF, Kaye M: Hemodialysis neutropenia and dialyzer reuse: role of the cleansing agent. Uremia Invest 8:17–20, 1984.

43. Rancourt M, Senger K, De Oreo P: Cellulosic membrane induced leukopenia after reprocessing with sodium hypochlorite. Trans Am Soc Artif Intern Organs 30:49–51, 1984.

44. Dorson W, Pizziconi V, Hyde G: Technical considerations in multiple use of dialyzers. In: Sadler J (ed) Proceedings of the national workshop on the reuse of consumables in hemodialysis. Kidney Disease Coalition, Washington DC 1983 pp 11–39.

45. Man NK, Lebkiri B, Polo P, De Sainte-Lorette E, Lemaire A, Funck-Brentano JL: Prevention of anti-N-like antibodies development with nonformaldehyde reuse procedure. Proc Dial Transplant Forum 10:18–21, 1980.
46. Berkseth R, Luehmann D, McMichael C, Keshaviah P, Kjellstrand C: Peracetic acid for reuse of hemodialyzers: clinical studies. Trans Am Soc Artif Intern Organs 30:270–275, 1984.
47. Petersen NJ, Carson LA, Favero MS: Bacterial endotoxin in new and reused hemodialyzers: a potential cause of endotoxemia. Trans Am Soc Artif Intern Organs 27:155–160, 1981.
48. Sigdell JE: New hollow-fiber dialyzers. Artif Organs 9:205–220, 1985.
49. Peterson NJ: Microbiologic hazards asociated with reuse of hemodialyzers. In: Sadler J (ed) Proceedings of the national workshop on the reuse of consumables in hemodialysis. Kidney Disease Coalition, Washington DC, 1983 pp 119–134.
50. Favero MS: Recommendations for water quality and sterilant elution. In: Deane N, Wineman RJ (eds) Seminar on reuse of hemodialyzers: automated and manual methods. National Nephrology Foundation, New York, 1984.
51. Petersen NJ, Carson LA, Doto IL, Aguero SM, Favero MS: Microbiologic evaluation of a new glutaraldehyde-based disinfectant for hemodialysis systems. Trans Am Soc Artif Intern Organs 28:287–290. 1982.
52. Wendt TM, Bell WM, Berry RF: Safety, efficacy, and performance of CIDEX dialyzer disinfectant for reprocessing hemodialyzers. AAMI Technology Assessment Report 10–85. Hemodialyzer reuse: issues and solutions. Association for the Advancement of Medical Instrumentation, Arlington VA, 1985, pp 26–31.
53. Wineman, RJ, Vogel RA, Bemis JA: A preliminary report on a comparative evaluation of sterilant/disinfectants for hemodialyzers reprocessing. AAMI Technical Assessment Report 10–85. Hemodialyzer reuse: issues and solutions. Association for the Advancement of Medical Instrumentation, Arlington VA, 1985, pp 32–34.
54. Hakim RM: Evaluation of the efficacy and safety of SPORICIDIN-HD for disinfecting new and reused dialyzers and hemodialysis machines. Dial Transplant 13:769–778, 1984.
55. De Palma JR: Clinical comparison of different cold sterilants for dialyzer reprocessing. Paper presented at the International Workshop on Hemodialyzer Reprocessing, 21 September 1984, Bad Homburg, FRG (to be published).
56. Moss A, Khakoo R, Shen SH, Whittier F: Dialyzer reprocessing decreases endotoxin reactivity of eluate from cuprophan membranes [abstr]. Am Soc Artif Intern Organs 14:25, 1985.
57. Pizziconi VB, Dorson WJ, Carson LA, Walsh SA, Brady RL, Cherill DA: Reuse, CUPROPHAN dialyzers, endotoxin contamination, and neutropenia. In: Sadler J (ed) Proceedings of the national workshop on reuse of consumables in hemodialysis. Kidney Disease Coalition, Washington DC, 1983, pp 72–91.
58. Bauer H, Brunner H, Franz HE: Experience with the disinfectant peroxyacetic acid (PES) for hemodialyzer reuse. Trans Am Soc Artif Intern Organs 29:662–665, 1983.
59. Buoncristiani U, Bianchi P, Barzi AM, Quintaliani G, Cozzari M, Carobi C: An ideal disinfectant for peritoneal dialysis. Int J Nephrol Urol Androl 1:45–48, 1980.
60. Pappalardo G, Tanner F: Evaluation of a disinfectant in accordance with Swiss standards. Drugs Exp Clin Res 9:109–113, 1983.
61. Lamperi S, Carozzi S, Icardi A, Trasforini D: An electrolytic chloroxidizer in nephrology: the reuse of dialyzers. Colloquia Med Santoriana 6:65–75, 1980.
62. Ciancione C, Naret C, Picot A, Poignet JL, Delons S, Man NK: Cutaneous hypersensitivity reactions to dialyzer extract and ethylene oxide in haemodialyzed patients [abstr]. Eur Dial Transplant Assoc, 1985, p 103.
63. Pizzaconi VB, Dorson WJ, Breillat J, Hyde GM, Aniuk LM, Walsh SA, Bland LA, Brady RL: Factors affecting complement activation and neutropenia during dialysis using cuprophane membranes. Am Soc Artif Intern Organs J 7:64–73, 1984.
64. Yamagami S, Niwa M, Kishimoto T, Umeda M, Tanaka S, Iwanaga S: Limulus positive substance in the CUPROPHANE membrane for hemodialysis [abstr]. Am Soc Artif Intern Organs 14:33, 1985.
65. Van Holder R: Two years experience with automated reprocessing of hemofilters and hemodialyzers. Paper presented at the International Workshop on Hemodialyzer Reprocessing, 21 September 1984, Bad Homburg, FRG (to be published).
66. Pitt AM, McDowell J, McElhinney S: Anticoagulant and kinetic effects on complement

activation [abstr]. Am Soc Artif Intern Organs 14:28, 1985.
67. Lewis KJ, Ward MK, Kerr DNS: Residual formaldehyde in dialyzers: quantity, location and effect of different methods of rinsing. Artif Organs 5:269–277, 1981.
68. Kaye M, Barber E, Gagnon R: Residual formaldehyde in new and reused dialyzers [abstr]. Am Soc Artif Intern Organs 14:32, 1985.
69. Keshaviah P, Leumann D, Ilstrup K: Particulate contamination of hemodialyzers [abstr]. Dial Transplant Forum 11:16, 1981.

3. SOLUTE AND WATER TRANSPORT AND STERILANT REMOVAL IN REUSED DIALYZERS

FRANK A. GOTCH

SOLUTE AND WATER TRANSPORT

Since variable decay of solute and water transport rates can be expected in reused dialyzers, it is essential that the magnitude of decay be predictable in an individual dialyzer prior to certification that it is suitable for reuse. Practical clinical reality further requires that this certification be based on an inexpensive and easily measured property of the reused dialyzer that can be quantitatively related to the transport capacity.

The overall rate of solute transport or net flux (N) in the dialyzer is a function of the overall transport coefficient (Ko), effective membrane area (A), and the appropriately defined mean concentration gradient ($\overline{\Delta C}$) as shown in equation 3.1:

$$N = Ko \ldots A \ldots \overline{\Delta C} \tag{3.1}$$

The Ko is a fundamental dialyzer physical constant and depends on membrane permeability, blood and dialysate channel geometry, and blood and dialysate flow distribution. Membrane fouling from protein deposition and blockage from clotting can result in decreased KoA and decreased N.

The ultrafiltration rate (QF) of the device is dependent on the hydraulic permeability constant of the membrane (kuf), membrane area, and mean transmembrane pressure ($\overline{TMP}$) as shown in equation 3.2:

$$QF = kuf \cdot A \cdot \overline{TMP} \tag{3.2}$$

Deane, Wineman, and Bemis (eds.): GUIDE TO REPROCESSING OF HEMODIALYZERS.
© 1986. Martinus Nijhoff Publishing. All rights reserved.

Decreased ultrafiltration capacity, kuf·A can result from decreased membrane permeability or effective area in reused dialyzers for the reasons given above.

Prediction of solute and water transport in individual reused dialyzers is thus ideally based on the demonstration that Ko, kuf, and A are dependent variables of an easily measured property of the reused device. The clinical parameters of interest are dialysance (D), clearance (K), and the overall ultrafiltration coefficient, which can be defined as KUF = kuf·A. The relationship between these clinical parameters and the more fundamental transport constants, K and kuf, can be determined from well-known transport equations [1].

Total effective membrane area is a critical parameter controlling solute transport (equation 3.1) and would be predicted to be a good property of the reused dialyzer to correlate with solute transport capacity. The only current dialyzer in which change in A can be easily measured is the hollow-fiber kidney (HFK). These devices have noncompliant blood compartments so that the priming volume before and after use is easily measured. It has been shown that hydraulic resistance to blood flow and volume of blood trapped in the fiber bundle both correlate closely with loss of priming volume in these devices [2, 3], indicating that whole fibers become plugged and area loss should thus be directly proportional to priming volume loss.

All parallel plate and coil geometry dialyzers have variably compliant blood compartments so that change in priming volume cannot be reliably measured. Consequently, other than actual measured clearances and ultrafiltration rates, there is no physical property that can be used to certify an individual device for reuse.

Two mechanisms have been proposed to result in decreased solute transport in the reprocessed hollow-fiber dialyzer. The first mechanism proposed was thrombus formation with occlusion of clotted fibers resulting in loss of effective membrane area [2–6]. This mechanism can be quantified by comparing the fiber bundle volume (FBV, ml) measured after reprocessing to the FBV measured prior to clinical use. The clearance of the reprocessed device can then be predicted from the loss of effective membrane area and the overall permeability–area product (KoA, ml/min) using standard transport equations.

More recently it has been proposed that the major mechanism resulting in decreased clearance is protein deposition on the membrane resulting in decreased membrane permeability to solute [7]. Study of this proposed mechanism has been pursued through in vitro measurements of dialyzer clearance and hydraulic permeability and empirical correlation of solute clearance to membrane hydraulic resistance, the reciprocal of hydraulic permeability [7].

Theoretical effect of thrombotic fiber occlusion on clearance

It is assumed that the magnitude of clotting can be directly measured from change in FBV and change in effective membrane area directly calculated from change in FBV [4]. A standard transport equation [1] can then be used to calculate predicted clearance in the reprocessed device in accordance with

$$K = \left[1 - e^{\frac{KoA}{QB}(1-\frac{QB}{QD})}\right] \bigg/ \left[\frac{QB}{QD} - e^{\frac{KoA}{QB}(1-\frac{QB}{QD})}\right] \tag{3.3}$$

where K = dialyzer clearance, ml/min; and QB and QD are blood and dialysate flow rates, ml/min.

Theoretical effect of protein deposition on clearance

In this case it is assumed that the membrane is thickened due to protein deposition, which results in decreased FBV due to reduced fiber ID, but not necessarily loss in area. This mechanism is postulated to reduce clearance primarily by increasing membrane resistance to solute transport. The change in membrane resistance to solute transport is assumed to be proportional to change in membrane hydraulic resistance and thus clearance in the reprocessed device is reported as a function of the hydraulic resistance [7].

The theoretical effects of this mechanism are more complex than the case where the mechanism is assumed to be only loss of area due to clotting. In the case of the protein deposition mechanism, change in clearance is predicted mechanistically from change in Ko resulting from increased membrane solute resistance. In the development that follows, it will be assumed that both mechanisms, protein deposition and area loss, can occur and that both are proportional to membrane hydraulic resistance. In this way an envelope of predicted clearances encompassing the entire spectrum from pure area loss to pure increased membrane resistance can be constructed as a function of membrane hydraulic resistance and compared with clinical data.

Assuming that change in membrane resistance to solute transfer (Rm, min/cm) is directly proportional to change in membrane hydraulic resistance (Rh, mmHg·Hr·ml^{-1}), the relation of Rm to Rh prior to clinical use is

$$Rmo = kRho \tag{3.4}$$

where k is a proportionality constant. After dialyzer reprocessing the relationship is

$$Rmt = Rmo + k\left[(Rht - Rho)(1 - B)\right] \tag{3.5}$$

where B is the fraction of change in Rh due to blocked fibers and area loss that increases Rh, but does not effect any change in Rm.

Combination of equations 3.4 and 3.5 and solution for Rmt results in

$$Rmt = Rmo\left[\frac{Rht}{Rho}(1 - B) + B\right] \tag{3.6}$$

Equation 3.6 describes the effect of $\triangle$Rh on Rm over a spectrum of B ranging from 0 to 1.

The ultrafiltration coefficient (KUF, ml·h^{-1}·mmHg^{-1}) is directly proportional to area in accordance with

$$KUF = kA \qquad (3.7)$$

where k is a proportionality constant.

Since Rh is the reciprocal of KUF, it follows that, prior to first use,

$$\frac{1}{Rho} = kAo \qquad (3.8)$$

and in the reprocessed dialyzer

$$\frac{1}{Rht} = kAo - k(Ao - At)B \qquad (3.9)$$

where B is the fraction of change in Rh due to blocked fibers and area loss with the assumption that this area is no longer available for ultrafiltration.

Combination of equations 3.8 and 3.9 and solution for At results in

$$At = Ao \left[1 - \frac{1}{B} (1 - \frac{Rho}{Rht}) \right] \qquad (3.10)$$

The total solute transport resistance (RT) is the sum of the blood (Rb), dialysate (Rd) and membrane (Rm) resistances and RT is the reciprocal of Ko. Thus it follows that, in the dialyzer prior to use,

$$KoAo = \frac{Ao}{Rmo + Rb + Rd} \qquad (3.11)$$

As discussed above, the values of A and Rm may be expected to be changed in the reprocessed dialyzer while Rb and Rd are expected to remain constant. By combining equations 3.6, 3.10, and 3.11, we can define KotAt in the reprocessed device from change in membrane hydraulic resistance in accordance with

$$KotAt = \frac{Ao \left[1 - \frac{1}{B} (1 - \frac{Rho}{Rht}) \right]}{Rmo \left[\frac{Rht}{Rho} (1 - B) + B \right] + Rb + Rd} \qquad (3.12)$$

Clinical data base for the FBV reuse criterion

There is a substantial data base relating clearance and ultrafiltration to FBV in the reprocessed dialyzer [2, 4–6]. It has been shown that urea and creatinine clearances in the reprocessed dialyzer can be predicted from FBV measurement and equation 3.3 with high-level precision. The data reported by Deane and Bemis [6] showed 95% confidence limits on urea and creatinine clearances predicted from FBV to be ± 12 and ± 13 ml/min, respectively, based on an average or generic initial FBV for the dialyzers

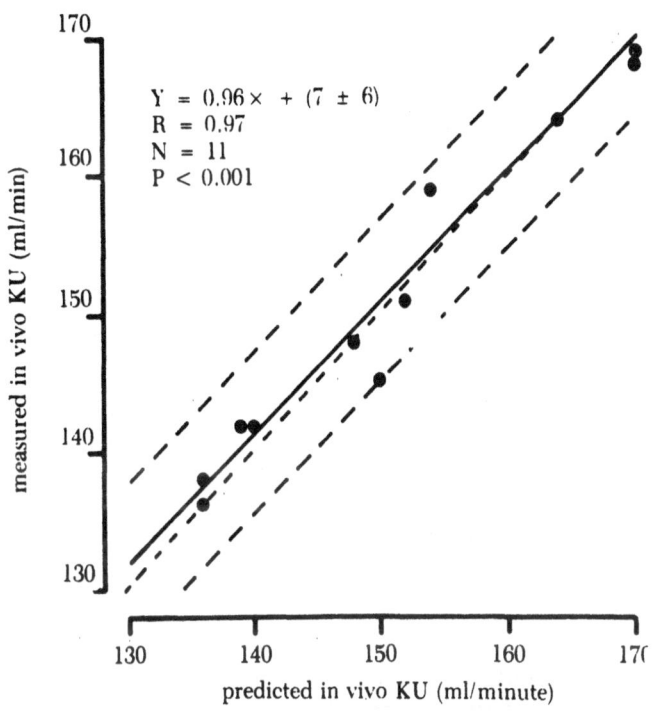

Figure 3-1. Correlation of measured end dialysis in vivo Ku to predicted Ku calculated from end-dialysis FBV and measured in vitro FBV and Ku prior to use. Reproduced with permission from *Hemodialyzer reuse: issues and solutions*, pp 38–40 (copyright 1985 by the Association for the Advancement of Medical Instrumentation, Arlington, VA).

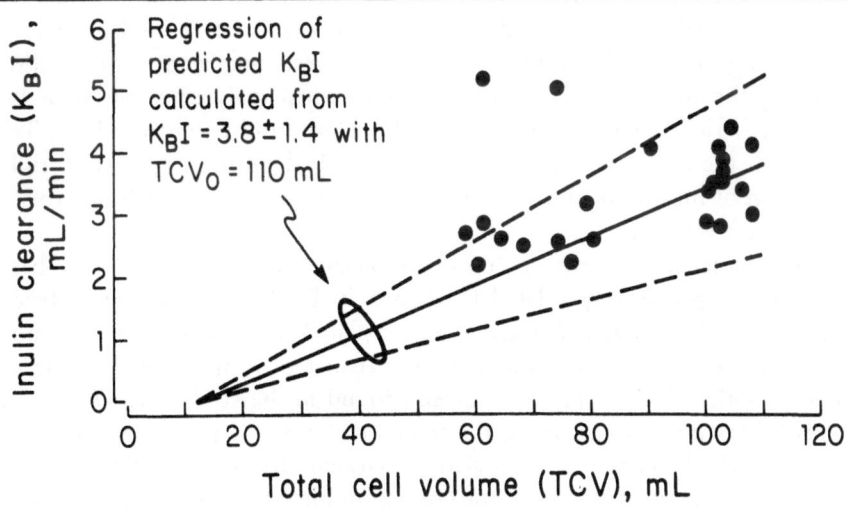

Figure 3-2. Comparison of measured and predicted inulin clearance as a function of TCV.

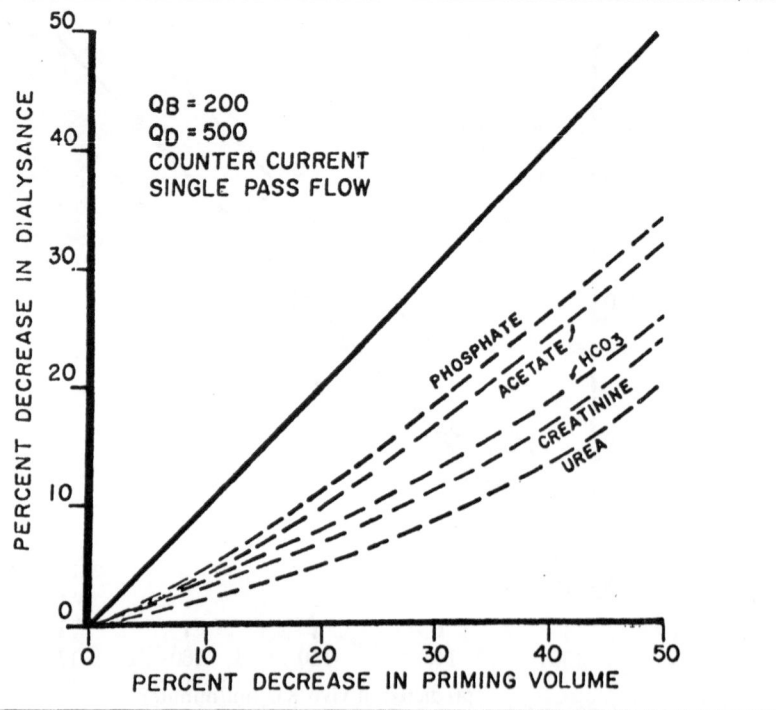

Figure 3-3. Calculated change in clearance as a function of decrease in priming volume for C-DAK 1.8 dialyzer. Reproduced, with permission, from Gotch [4].

studied. We have recently measured the urea clearance in vivo in reused dialyzers at the beginning and end of dialysis. In this study, in vitro urea clearance, FBV and effective area were measured prior to first use for each device and FBV was measured at the end of each dialysis and after each reprocessing. The predicted in vivo clearances were calculated from equation 3.3 using the measured KoAo for each individual dialyzer rather than the average generic value for the device as in the Deane and Bemis data base. The results of these studies shown in figure 3-1 demonstrate a very tight correlation of measured to predicted in vivo clearance to ± 6 ml/min at 95% confidence level.

Larger molecular weight or "middle molecule" clearances also have been shown to be predictably related to change in FBV in the reused dialyzer. Farrell et al. [5] showed that area loss calculated from decrease in vitamin-B12 clearance agreed well with area loss calculated from change in priming volume (within 1.2%). The relationship found in the studies by Deane and Bemis [6] for inulin clearance in the reused dialyzer is depicted in figure 3-2. The two asterisked data points deviating markedly from the predicted regression were single measurements not done in duplicate and hence less reliable. The data in figure 3-2 indicate that inulin clearance in the reused dialyzer can

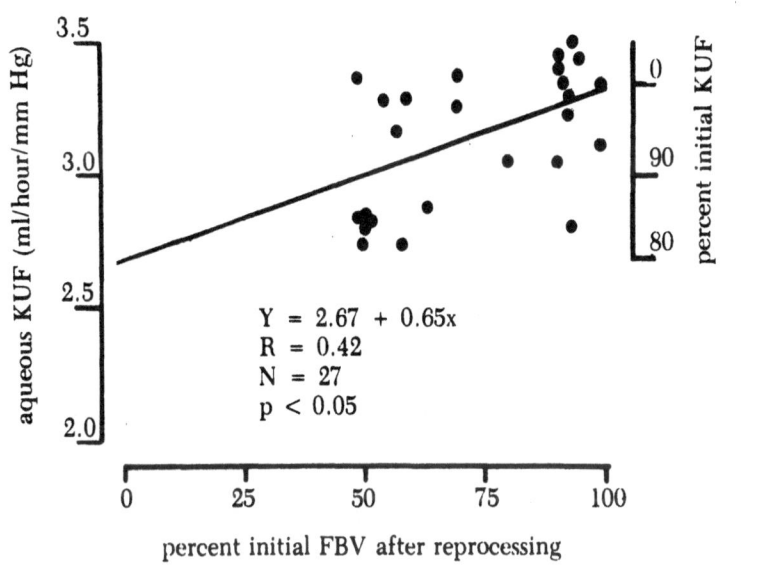

Figure 3-4. Relationship between aqueous in vitro KUF and FBV. Reproduced with permission from *Hemodialyzer reuse: issues and solutions*, pp 38−40 (Copyright 1985 by the Association for the advancement of Medical Instrumentation, Arlington, VA).

be predicted with confidence from measured change in FBV.

There will be a family of curves describing clearance of individual solutes as area is lost during reuse as shown in figure 3-3 for a typical hollow-fiber kidney [4]. The curves in figure 3-3 are interpreted to show that the loss in priming volume should be ≤20% for certification of an individual dialyzer for reuse. With this constraint, the loss in dialysance of all solutes shown will be quite small and range from 4% to 11%. As the priming volume loss increases above 20%, the acetate and bicarbonate curves begin to separate with greater loss in acetate than bicarbonate dialysance due to the lower acetate Ko. This could have a significant impact on acid−base balance since correction with acetate dialysis is dependent on a small difference between quite high rates of acetate flux into and bicarbonate flux out of the patient. The proportionally greater loss of acetate dialysance beyond a 20% loss in priming volume could result in poorer correction of metabolic acidosis.

The loss of vitamin B12 and inulin clearance would be nearly equal to the identity line in figure 3-3 due to the high membrane resistance. If dialysis therapy were prescribed as a linear function of these solute clearances, treatment time would have to be increased in direct proportion to loss in priming volume in reused dialyzers. However, there is no generally accepted evidence that dialyzer vitamin B12 and inulin clearances are determinants of the dialysis prescription.

In contrast to the highly predictable relationship of clearance to FBV, the

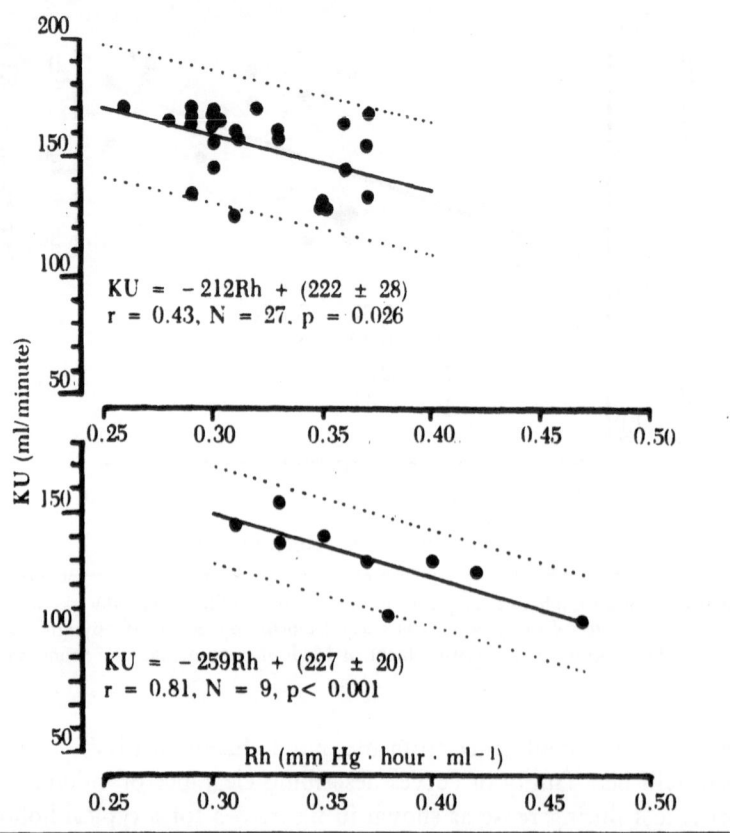

Figure 3-5. Empirical correlations of urea clearance (Ku) to membrane hydraulic resistance (Rh) in reprocessed dialyzers.

in vitro aqueous KUF is very loosely correlated to FBV. The relationship found by Deane and Bemis [6] is shown in figure 3-4 and, although there is a significant relationship ($p<0.05$), there is a great deal of scatter in the data. It is also clearly apparent that the in vitro KUF does not decrease in direct proportion with decrease in FBV and effective area. The slope is shallow and the regression extrapolates to a KUF = 2.67 ml/h/mmHg when FBV = 0. This intercept value is 80% of the in vitro KUF prior to first use and demonstrates that thrombus material occluding fibers is highly porous with high hydraulic permeability. However, this cannot be interpreted to mean that the occluded fibers will have a similar high hydraulic permeability in the reprocessed dialyzer in vivo. Although the thrombus-occluded fibers are permeable to water, a rapid buildup or protein concentration in the luminal fluid can be predicted when plasma is ultrafiltered in vivo. (F. Gotch, unpublished observations). The resulting increase in oncotic pressure will result in rapid cessation of ultrafiltration in the occluded fibers and in vivo KUF will

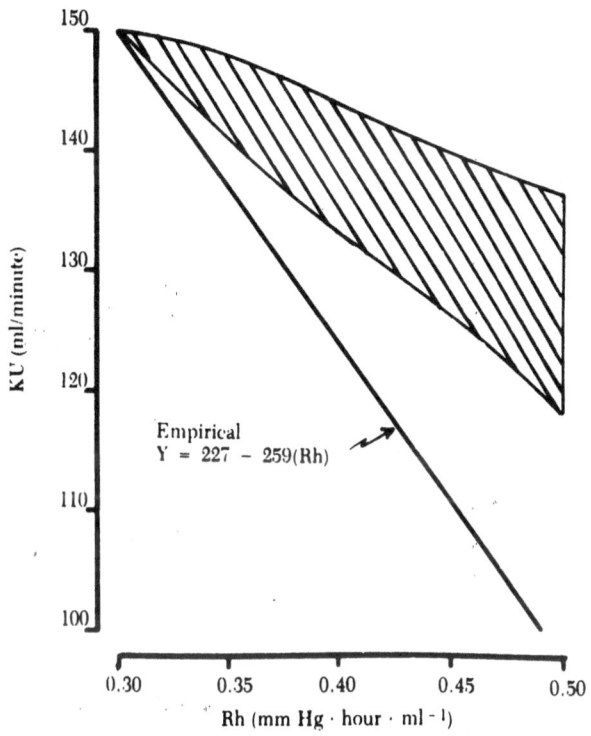

Figure 3-6. Comparison of empirical correlation of Ku with Rh to predicted correlation based on mechanistic considerations.

decrease in direct proportion with decrease in FBV and effective area. During reprocessing with reverse ultrafiltration the protein buildup is washed out and a high aqueous in vitro ultrafiltration coefficient is restored in the occluded fibers.

Clinical data base for the Rh reuse criterion

Studies correlating urea, creatinine, and vitamin-B12 clearances to membrane hydraulic resistance have also been reported [7]. The regressions of urea clearance on Rh shown in figure 3-5 are calculated from data reported by Dorson et al. [7] and Deane and Bemis [6]. It is apparent that there is a significant relationship of urea clearance to Rh for both sets of data but the 95% confidence limits on the predicted clearance are ± 20 to ± 28 ml/min, approximately twice the confidence limits for the regression of urea clearance on FBV in the reprocessed dialyzer.

The urea and creatinine clearances in the reprocessed dialyzer correlate highly with those predicted from KotAt determined from change in A calculated from change in FBV. This provides strong support of the concept that the mechanism of clearance loss is due to fiber occlusion and resultant

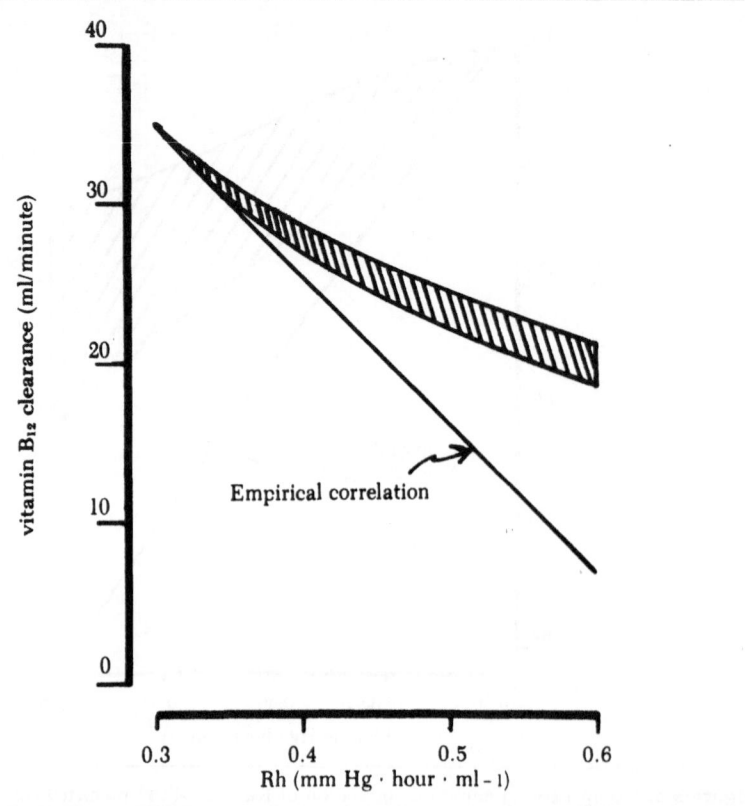

Figure 3-7. Comparison of empirical and predicted correlations of KB12 to Rh.

loss of effective area. It is instructive to compare the empirical relationships reported [7] between clearance and Rh with the relationship predicted from mechanistic consideration of protein deposition on the fiber luminal surface and/or fiber occlusion with area loss. In this analysis it is assumed that change in Rm and A is directly proportional to change in Rh due to protein deposition or fiber occlusion as in the development above of equations 3.4 through 3.12.

The empirical regression of urea clearance (KU) on Rh shown in figure 3-6 is calculated from the data reported [6]. The regression envelope depicted was calculated from equation 3.3 and 3.12 with B varied from 0 (pure protein deposition, envelope upper bound) to 1.0 (pure fiber occlusion, envelope lower bound). The envelope was constructed using the following typical Travenol 1211 dialyzer transport parameters: KoAo = 350 ml/min, corresponding to Rh = 0.30; A = 12,000 cm^2; Ko = 0.02917 cm/min; Rmo = 13.7 min/cm, Rb + Rd = 20.6 min/cm.

The results in figure 3-6 show that the empirical correlation of KU to Rh falls well below the mechanistically predicted envelope based on either pro-

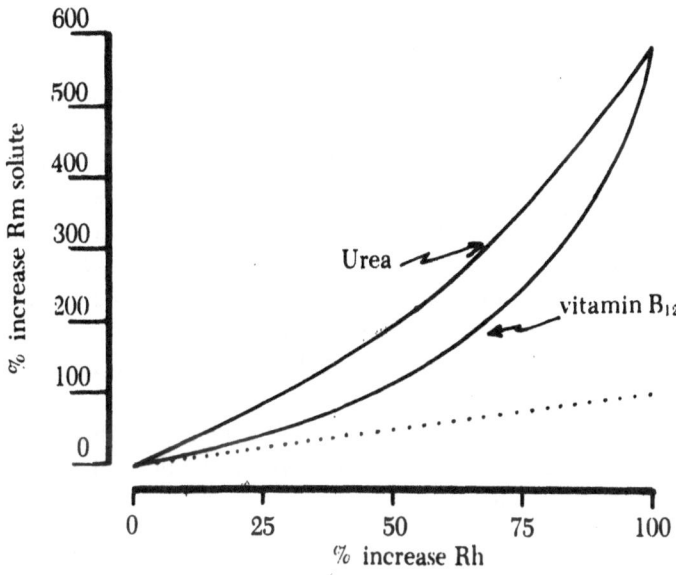

Figure 3-8. Increase in membrane solute resistance compared with increase in hydraulic resistance.

tein deposition or fiber occlusion with the assumption that both of these
mechanisms can be quantified from measurement of membrane hydraulic
resistance. This will be discussed further below.

The empirical regression of vitamin–B12 clearance (KB12) on Rh calculated
from the reported data [7] is shown in figure 3-7 with a regression envelope
predicted from mechanistic considerations as in figure 3-6. The transport
parameters used for the KB12 calculations were: KoAo = 40 ml/min, corresponding to Rh = 0.30; A = 12,000 cm^2; Ko = 0.0033 cm/min; Rmo = 259
min/cm; Rb + Rd = 44 min/cm.

The results in figure 3-7 also show that the empirical regression of KB12
on Rh falls well below the mechanistically predicted regression envelope. In
the case of vitamin B12, the lower bound on the regression envelope corres-
ponds to pure fiber occlusion and area loss, the opposite with respect to KU,
due to the large fraction of total resistance contributed by the membrane in
the case of vitamin B12. The location of the empirical regression well below
the lower bound of the envelope suggests that area loss is considerably
underestimated from measured change in Rh.

The much steeper decrease in KU and KB12 as functions of Rh compared
with the predicted envelopes in figures 3-6 and 3-7 might result from Rm
increasing more rapidly than Rh with membrane protein deposition. The
percent increases in Rm for urea and vitamin B12 were calculated for the
empirical regressions in figures 3-6 and 3-7 using the transport parameters
listed above. The results are shown in figure 3-8 where they are plotted

against percent increase in Rh. The curves in figure 3-8 are not reassuring that the mechanism for clearance loss in the reprocessed dialyzer is membrane protein deposition. The curves are nonlinear and there is no a priori reason to expect a nonlinear increase in solute resistance as the membrane is thickened. The Rm increase for urea is substantially greater than for vitamin B12 until a 100% increase in Rh is reached, at which point the increased Rm for both solutes is equal and six times the increase in Rh. It is not reasonable to expect a protein layer to result in greater increase in Rm for urea with molecular weight 60 daltons compared with vitamin B12 with molecular weight of 1350 daltons. It is also not reasonable to expect a severalfold greater increase in solute resistance compared with hydraulic resistance. It is well known that in conventional cellulosic hollow-fiber dialyzers the in vivo KUF on first use is 10%−20% less than the in vitro value while the in vivo KU is virtually identical to the in vitro value. Thus it is difficult to visualize a mechanism whereby membrane−protein interaction would result in a sixfold greater increase in Rm than in Rh.

Reconciliation of the FBV and Rh criteria for reuse

Clearance loss in the reprocessed dialyzer is highly predictable from change in FBV and its direct correlate, area loss. This strongly supports area loss as the only significant mechanism resulting in loss of clearance. In contrast, because of the high in vitro hydraulic permeability of thrombus, the in vitro KUF is loosely correlated with FBV and decreases much less rapidly than effective area decreases with fiber occlusion (see figure 3-4). The inverse of KUF, Rh, can thus be confidently predicted to underestimate the magnitude of area loss and to quantify area loss less precisely in the reprocessed device. The under-estimation of area loss by the Rh parameter would result in the steeper clearance loss as a function of Rh in figures 3-6 and 3-7 compared with the predicted envelopes and the severalfold greater apparent increases in Rm relative to Rh in figure 3-8. The much looser correlation of Rh to effective area compared with FBV and effective area would result in the two fold greater standard deviation on clearance predicted from Rh shown in figure 3-5.

Summary

(1) Decreased solute transport in reused dialyzers is due to fiber occlusion by thrombus and resultant loss of effective membrane area. (2) Solute transport capacity can therefore be predicted from change in priming volume (FBV), which relates directly to area loss. (3) Precision for urea clearance predicted in the reprocessed dialyzer from generic KoA reference values is ± 12 ml/min and increases to ± 6 ml/min with individualized KoA reference values. (4) The aqueous in vitro KUF grossly underestimates area loss due to the high hydraulic permeability of thrombus. (5) There is a loose empirical correlation of urea clearance to in vitro membrane hydraulic resistance, but the standard

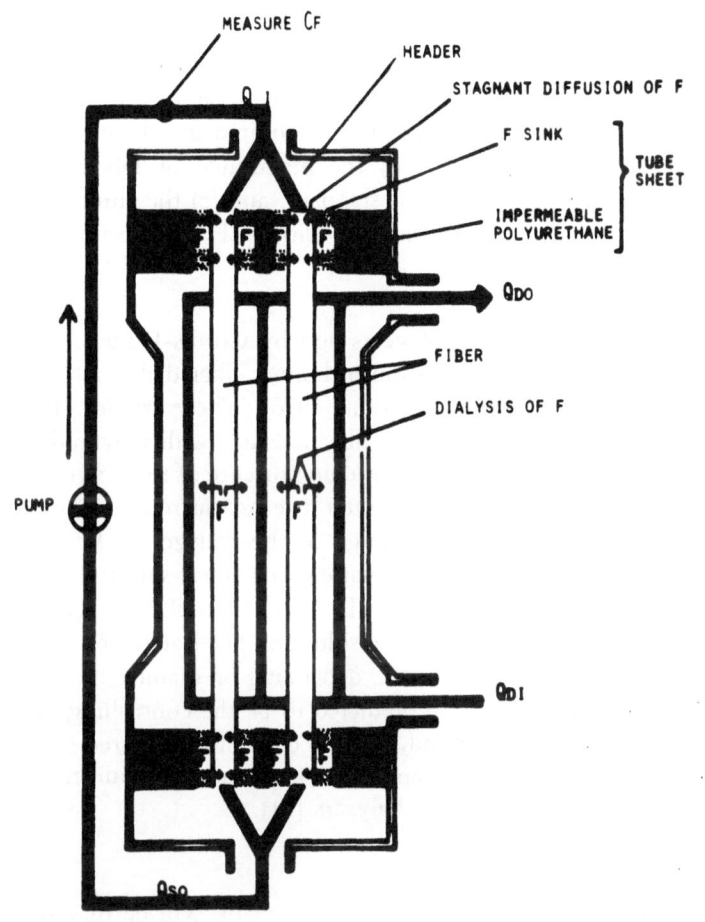

Figure 3-9. The formaldehyde (F) sink in hollow-fiber dialyzers. Reproduced, with permission, from Gotch and Keen [11].

deviation is two times greater than the correlation of clearance to FBV. Therefore, in virto measurement of membrane hydraulic resistance is a less reliable method for certification of a reprocessed dialyzer for clinical use compared with measurement of FBV. (6) The decrease in FBV should be less than or equal to 20% for certification of the dialyzer for reuse with respect to solute and water transport. If reuse is practiced with greater than 20% area loss, there should be appropriate increases in blood flow rate and/or treatment time to compensate for decreases in solute and water transport.

STERILANT REMOVAL

Formaldehyde (F) is the most widely used sterilant for processing the reused dialyzer (RD). There are both concerns and controversy regarding safe residual F levels in the dialyzer. Recommendations in the literature for safe F concentrations (CF) in the final rinse solution range from 2 ppm [8] to 10 ppm [9] and the state of California has tentatively mandated <1 ppm [10]. The kinetics of F removal from the RD will be reviewed here for the purposes of determining (a) rinsing times required to achieve specified rinse CF values at 95% confidence, (b) the magnitude of rebound CF to be expected if the rinse solution is left stagnant, and (c) the cumulative F doses infused during dialysis after rinsing to various CF levels prior to dialysis.

The formaldehyde sink

Studies were done a number of years ago by Cordis-Dow Corporation to determine the site of F sequestration in hollow-fiber dialyzers (Cordis-Dow Corporation, personal communication, 1976). These studies showed that, during dialyzer fabrication, cellulosic fiber interacts with polyurethane potting material that partially inhibits the hardening or cure of the polyurethane. The result is a thin film or cuff of polyurethane gel surrounding each fiber as depicted in figure 3-9. During storage of the dialyzer in F, the F slowly diffuses into this gel layer, which becomes a chemical sink for F. During the rinsing procedure, F must be leached (L) out of the sink by stagnant diffusion through the fiber walls into the rinse solution. The size of the sink might be expected to vary in different devices, depending on manufacturing processes. Further, the sink size would be predicted to be the controlling factor determining rinsing time, CF rebound, and the dose of F delivered to the pateint. Consequently, the tube sheet F sink is the key kinetic parameter determining residual F levels in hollow-fiber dialyzers [11].

Formaldehyde kinetic model

The rate of F diffusion or leaching from the sink will be maximized if the rinse CF is minimized. Since F dialysance is high, low rinse CF can best be achieved by recirculation of rinse solution in the blood compartment with single pass flow through the dialysate compartment as shown in figure 3-9. Mass balance of F in the blood loop under these conditions is described by

$$V\frac{dc}{dt} = L(t) - KC \tag{3.13}$$

where L, mg/min, is a function of t, min; K is F clearance, L/min; C is F concentration, mg/L or ppm; and V is L.

Solution of equation 3.13 results in

$$C_t = C_o e^{\frac{-Kt}{V}} + \frac{\bar{L}}{K}(1 - e^{\frac{-Kt}{V}}) \tag{3.14}$$

which, when solved for $\bar{L}$, yields

$$\bar{L} = \frac{Ct - Coe^{-\overline{Kt}}}{1 - e^{-\overline{Kt}}} K \tag{3.15}$$

The rate of leaching from the sink, L, is not constant and decreases as a function of t as the sink becomes depleted during the recirculating rinse procedure. Consequently mean values, $\bar{L}$, can be determined over short intervals by measuring CF every 5 min during recirculation and computing $\bar{L}$ for the midpoint of each 5-min interval.

Rinsing procedure

The recirculating rinse should be preceded by draining the dialysate compartment and establishment of single pass water flow through the compartment at 500 ml/min and 37°C and continued throughout the rinse procedure. The blood compartment is flushed with 700 ml saline single pass at 200 ml/min. Immediately after flush, the blood loop is closed and recirculation started at 400 ml/min. To establish the CF profile, samples for F measurement are taken from the venous blood line at the start of recirculation (t0) and every 5 min during rinsing. At the end of rinsing, blood and dialysate compartment flows are stopped and the system left stagnant to evaluate rebound CF. At the end of a specified stagnant interval, the blood lines are disconnected and the blood compartment solution blow out and analyzed to determine rebound CF. Formaldehyde can be measured spectrophotometrically using the acetyl acetone method [12]. The clearance of F is virtually identical to urea clearance of the dialyzer.

Calculations

The initial leaching rate ($\overline{LO}$ or $\overline{L2.5}$) is taken as the mean value at 2.5 min of recirculation calculated from equation 3.3 using the 0- and 5-min CF values. The dependence of $\overline{L2.5}$ on storage F concentration can be examined by linear regression analysis in accordance with

$$\overline{L2.5} = (a1 \pm 2SD) + b1(SF) \tag{3.16}$$

where a1 is the intercept, SD is standard deviation, b1 is slope, and SF is storage F concentration, %

As described above, mean $\overline{Lt}$ values are determined every 5 min during recirculation. The decay in $\bar{L}$ is best fitted to a power function of t and therefore analyzed, after logarithmic transformation, in accordance with

$$\frac{\overline{LT}}{\overline{L2.5}} = 10^{(a2 \pm 2SD)} \cdot t^{b2} \tag{3.17}$$

The rebound CF can be calculated from the measured $\bar{L}$ during the last 5 min of rinsing, the duration of the stagnant phase (t) and the volume of the blood compartment of the dialyzer (V) in accordance with

$$\text{rebound CF} = \frac{\overline{L \cdot t}}{V} \tag{3.18}$$

This expression can be expected to overestimate rebound CF greatly because the rate of diffusion out of the sink will rapidly decrease as CF increases locally in the stagnant rinse solution. However, it can be anticipated that a reproducible empirical relationship can be found between measured and calculated rebound CF reflecting the magnitude of F sink remaining the fixed stagnant diffusion geometry.

The rinse solution CF profiles (M+2SD) as a function of recirculation rinse time can be calculated for any dialyzer type using the constants determined for equations 3.16 and 3.17, which, when combined with equation 3.14, result in

$$Ct\pm 2SD) = Coe^{\frac{-Kt}{V}} + \frac{al+2SD) + bl(SF)\ 10^{(a2\pm 2SD)} \cdot t^{b2}}{K}(1-e^{\frac{-Kt}{V}} \tag{3.19}$$

Equation 3.19 can be solved numerically to calculate the rinse CF profiles for any dialyzer evaluated.

The cumulative dose of F (D) infused into the patient during dialysis is determined by the total amount of F leached from the sink during dialysis subsequent to rinsing and will be given by

$$D = \int_{0}^{td} L\ dt \tag{3.20}$$

This expression can be numerically integrated over the length of dialysis using the dialyzer leaching profile with t0 corresponding to rinse times required to achieve CF values of 10, 5, and 1 ppm prior to initiating dialysis.

Kinetically determined leaching rates for typical hollow-fiber dialyzers are shown in figure 3-10. A significant correlation between $\overline{L2.5}$ and storage F concentration can be seen (figure 3.10A). The leaching rate decreased as a highly predictable function of t as shown in figure 3-10B.

The results of typical rebound studies are shown in figure 3-11, where the data is expressed as the rate of rebound, ppm/min. There is a highly reproducible relationship between measured rebound CF and the value calculated from equation 3.18. The slope of 0.29 confirms the anticipation that equation 3.18 will overestimate rebound greatly, but that a predictable relationship will be found.

The F concentration profiles during rinsing (M±2SD) are calculated from kinetic data for the 1211 and 1511 dialyzers and shown in figure 3-12, where measured data points are also shown. The concentration profile is calculated for 1.5% F storage concentration.

The curves in figure 3-12 show that, to achieve maximum rinse CF values of 10, 5, 2, and 1 ppm, the required rinsing times are 5, 9, 15, and 24 min,

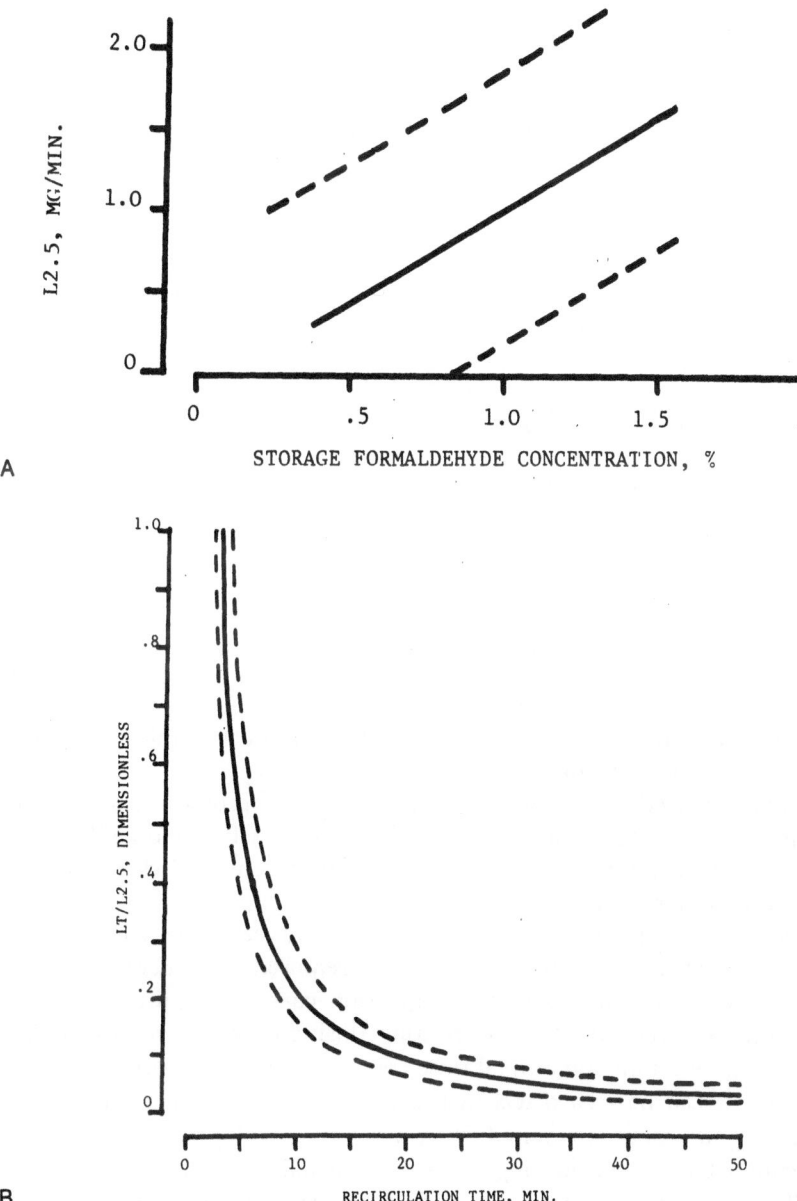

Figure 3-10. Results of kinetic studies of formaldehyde removal from Travenol 1211 and 1511 dialyzers.

    A. The correlation of initial formaldehyde leaching rate with the storage formaldehyde concentration.
    $Y = 1.15 \times -0.14 \pm 0.85.$ $R = 0.75.$ $P = 0.035$

    B. The ratio of leaching rate at time T, L_T, to the initial leaching rate, $L_{2.5}$, with recirculation time.
    $L_T/L_{2.5} = [10^{0.5894 \pm 0.1224}] \, T - 1.2648.$
    $R = 0.972, \, P < 0.001.$

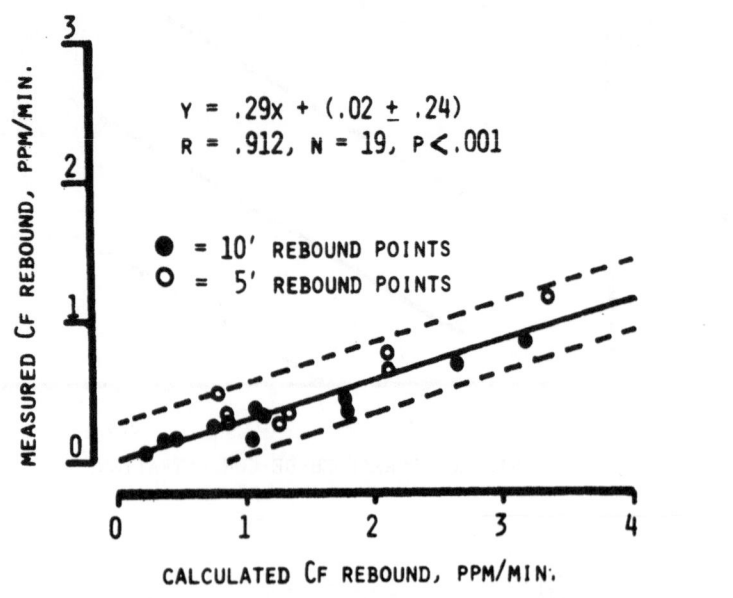

Figure 3-11. Comparison of actual rebound of formaldehyde concentration (CF) to that calculated from kinetics. Reproduced, with permission, from Gotch and Keen [11].

respectively. The mean rinse CF will be less than 2 ppm at 10 min respectively for the 1211 and 1511 dialyzers.

The curves labeled NS in figure 3-12 depict the CF profiles calculated for the device if there were no sink, i.e., L = 0. The rinse CF would fall below 1 ppm in less than 5 min of recirculation due to the high F clearance and small-volume blood loop.

It should be emphasized that these washout curves are based on 1.5% storage concentration and the rinsing time required will increase as the storage concentration increases. The regression curves in figure 3-13 were used to compute a family of curves relating rinsing time required to storage concentrations as a function of final rinse concentration with results shown in figure 3-13. It can be seen that a final concentration of 5 ppm will require ~15 min but, if 1 ppm is required, the rinsing time will increase to 45 min.

The cumulative patient loading doses of F calculated as a function of final rinse CF are shown in figure 3-14. Both the maximum and mean doses are calculated and can be compared with the California Occupational Safety and Health Agency (CAL-OSHA) standard for a safe level of inhaled F. The curves in figure 3-14 show that the maximal loading doses the patient would occasionally experience decrease from 14 to 8.5 mg as CF decreases from 10 to 1 ppm. The mean doses, which would determine the long-term patient F loading, are reduced very little, from 5.5 to 3.0 mg, when maximum CF is reduced from 10 to 1 ppm.

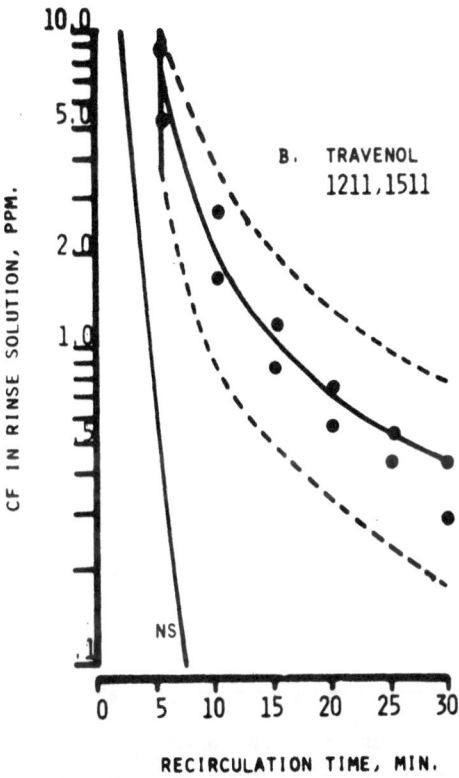

Figure 3-12. Formaldehyde concentration profiles (M±2SD) during recirculation rinse after storage in 1.5% formaldehyde. Lines *NS* show expected profile if there were no sink for formaldehyde in tube sheets. Reproduced, with permission, from Gotch and Keen [11].

The F kinetic model provides a method to quantify the magnitude of F sink which determines residual F levels in hollow-fiber dialyzers. The model can be used to guide studies to predict rinsing time reliably, rebound rate, and cumulative patient F load during dialysis for any specified dialyzer type and targeted final rinse CF.

The two major concerns regarding F toxicity are carcinogenesis and anti-N-like antibody (ANAb) formation. Carcinogenic risk would be expected to be related to cumulative F dose. The cumulative F dose required to produce nasal cancer in rats when extrapolated to humans would be 575 mg/week for 12 months or a total of 1500 mg F [13]. It would require 35 years of dialysis to reach this level of cumulative exposure with final rinse CF 10 ppm and 64 years with CF 1 ppm. There is no evidence of carcinogenesis reported in the literature with intravenous administration of F, which further enhances the disparity between the rat nasal carcinoma producing doses of F and the very small exposures in dialysis.

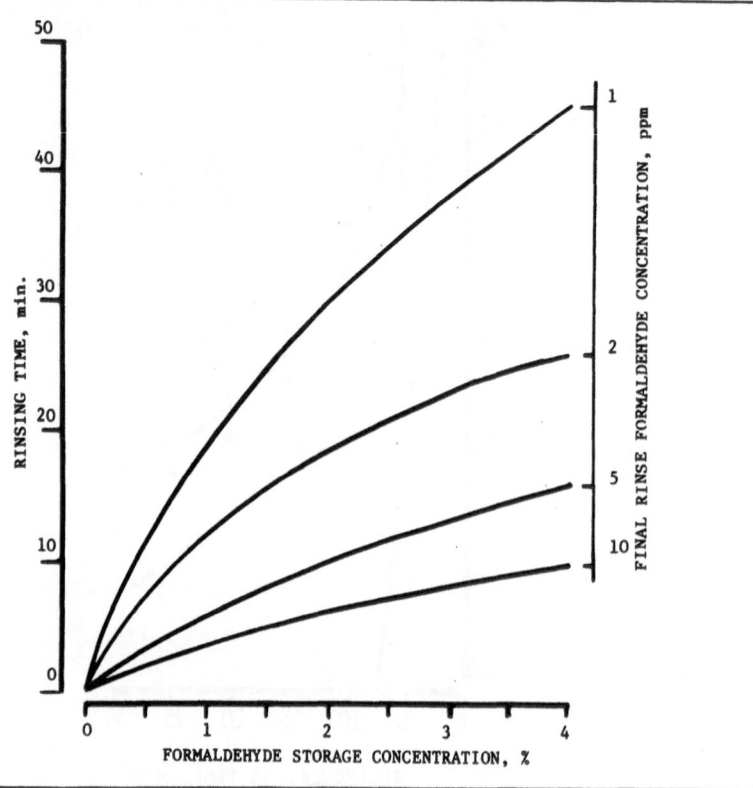

Figure 3-13. Rinsing time requirements as a function of sterilant storage concentration.

Formaldehyde has been used as urinary antiseptic for 90 years as methen-amine, which decomposes and liberates F at low pH. It can be calculated that with 4.0 g methenamine per day and 30% decomposition in acid gastric juice as much as 1500 mg F could be formed in the stomach and absorbed [14]. The bladder steady-state F concentrations reach 100–200 ppm with methenamine therapy. Recently F releasing agents have been used with considerable success in severe peritonitis [15].

In comparison to the level of F doses required to produce cancer ex-perimentally and the doses administered therapeutically in medicine, the small residual levels in dialyzers with final rinse CF <10 ppm would appear to pose a truly negligible risk for carcinogenesis.

The only established parenteral toxicity of F in humans is ANAb forma-tion. Lewis et al. reported a 30% incidence of ANAb in patients with mean final rinse CF of 8 ppm, range 3–13 [8]. Koch et al. found a similar incidence of ANAb with mean CF of 7 ppm, range 0.3–108 ppm [9]. Lewis et al. reported zero incidence ANAb with CF of 0.5–1 ppm and Koch et al. found ANAb disappeared when F reuse was eliminated. Lewis et al. recommended a maximum CF of 2 ppm while Koch et al. recommended 10 ppm; however,

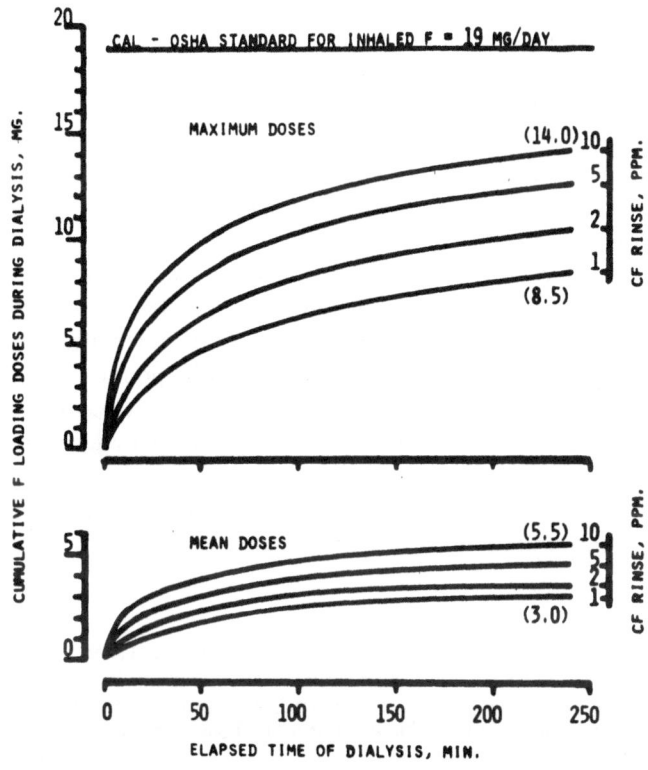

Figure 3-14. Cumulative mean and maximum formaldehyde loading doses during dialysis as a function of maximal final concentration of formaldehyde in rinse solution, calculated for SCE kidneys. Reproduced, with permission, from Gotch and Keen [11].

CF was not precisely controlled in either of these retrospective studies. In vitro studies by Koch et al. showed a minimum CF of 10 ppm was required for ANAb activity with NN cells and 50 ppm for MM cells [9]. (See chapter 9 for further details.)

In view of these data showing clinical ANAb formation with CF 7−8 ppm (and maximum values 13−108 ppm), it would seem quite reasonable to recommend a maximum CF <5 ppm, which would result in mean CF ≃ 2 ppm (see figure 3-12). This would require about 10-min rinse times for most hollow-fiber dialyzers stored in 1.5% F. A standard calling for maximum CF <1 ppm would appear to be too stringent in the light of scientific data available and would require rinsing times of up to 25 min in typical dialyzers stored in 1.5% F.

New sterilants

All water-soluble sterilants would be expected to diffuse into the tube sheet sink at a rate inversely proportional to the molecular weight of the sterilant. The long storage time results in substantial tube sheet uptake, which then must be removed rapidly during rinsing, and the rate at which sterilant diffuses out of the tube sheet during rinsing is also inversely proportional to molecular weight. On these grounds, formaldehyde should be the easiest to remove because its molecular weight is only 30 daltons whereas the new sterilants are larger. Sporicidin is comprised of glutaraldehyde and sodium phenate with molecular weights of 100–120 daltons while for peracetic acid the molecular weight is ~75. Thus these agents would be expected to be removed more slowly during rinsing.

The residual concentration of sterilant will be a function of both storage concentration and leaching kinetics during rinsing and at present there is little information to quantify these relationships for glutaraldehyde, sodium phenate, and peracetic acid. In this context it can also be pointed out that it may take a long time to uncover potential toxicity at low concentration of sterilants. It would not have been predicted that formaldehyde would result in anti-N antibodies at concentrations of 10 ppm in the rinse solution. Thus it is difficult to predict what clinical problems may appear with other sterilants over the low concentration range to be encountered.

REFERENCES

1. Sargent J, Gotch F: Principles and biophysics of dialysis. In: Drukker W, Parsons F, Maher J (eds). Replacement of renal function by dialysis. Martinus Nijhoff, Boston, 1983, pp 53–97.
2. Gotch F, Lipps B, Weaver J, Brandes J, Rosin J, Sargent J, Oja P: Chronic hemodialysis with the hollow fiber artificial kidney (HFAK). Trans Am Soc Artif Intern Organs 15:87–96, 1969.
3. Gotch F, Sargent J, Keen M, Holmes G, Teisinger C: Development and long term clinical evaluation of a thromboresistant hollow fiber kidney (HFK). Trans Am Soc Artif Intern Organs 18:135–145, 1972.
4. Gotch F: Mass transport in reused dialyzers. Proc Clin Dial Transplant Forum 10:81–85, 1980.
5. Farrell P, Eschbach J, Vizzo J, Babb L: Hemodialyzer reuse: estimation of area loss from clearance data. Kidney Int 5:466–450, 1974.
6. Deane N, Bemis J: Multiple use of hemodialyzers: final report to the National Institute of Arthritis, Diabetes and Digestive and Kidney Disease, contract NO1-AM-9-2214, pp 53–64, June 1981.
7. Dorson W, Pizziconi V, Hyde G: Technical considerations in multiple use of dialyzers. In: Sadler J (ed) Proceedings of the national workshop on the reuse of consumables in hemodialysis. Kidney Disease Coalition, Baltimore, 1983, pp 11–39.
8. Lewis KJ, Dewar PJ, Ward MK, Kerr DNS: Formation of anti-N-like antibodies in dialysis patients: effect of different methods of dialyzer rinsing to remove formaldehyde. Clin Nephrol 15:39–43, 1981.
9. Koch KM, Frei U, Fassbinder W: Hemolysis and anemia in anti-N-like antibody positive hemodialysis patients. Trans Am Soc Artif Intern Organs 24:709–713, 1978.
10. Draft regulations for dialyzer reuse. Food and Drug Branch, Department of Health Services, State of California, 1983.
11. Gotch F, Keen M: Formaldehyde kinetics in reused dialyzers. Trans Am Soc Artif Intern Organs 29:396–401, 1983.
12. Nash T: The colorimetric estimation of formaldehyde by means of the Hantzsch reaction. Biochem J 55:416–421, 1953.
13. Swenberg JA, Kerns WD, Mitchell RJ, Gralla, EJ, Pavkov KL: Induction of squamous cell carcinoma of the rat nasal cavity by inhalation exposure to formaldehyde vapor. Cancer Res 40:3398–3402, 1980.
14. Sande MA, Mandell GL: Antimicrobial agents: general considerations. In: Gilman AG,

Goodman LS, Gilman A (eds) Pharmacologic basis of therapeutics. Macmillan, New York, 1980, pp 1080–1105.

15. Browne MK, MacKenzie M, Doyle PJ: A controlled trial of taurolin in established bacterial peritonitis. Surg Gynecol Obstet 146:721–724, 1978.

4. MICROBIOLOGIC PRINCIPLES APPLIED TO REPROCESSING HEMODIALYZERS

MARTIN S. FAVERO

LEE A. BLAND

This chapter discusses important microbiologic considerations of dialyzer reuse. The terms *sterilization* and *disinfection* are defined especially in the context of dialyzer reuse, and microbiologic guidelines are described that are applied to water used to prepare dialysis fluid in contradistinction to water employed for rinsing dialyzers and preparing chemical germicide solutions in dialyzer reuse programs. Guidelines pertaining to bacterial endotoxin and chemicals in waters also are discussed.

DEFINITIONS

CDC activities in dialysis-associated diseases

The Centers for Disease Control (CDC) has the responsibility for investigating outbreaks of dialysis-associated diseases as well as formulating guidelines for the control of these diseases. The CDC collaborates with the National Institutes of Health, the Food and Drug Administration, the Health Care Finance Administration (HCFA), and with professional societies such as Renal Physicians Association and the Association for the Advancement of Medical Instrumentation. In cooperation with the HCFA, the CDC conducts an annual surveillance of dialysis-associated diseases in chronic hemodialysis centers in the United States [1]. Information is obtained on a variety of dialysis-associated diseases ranging from incidence and prevalence of viral hepatitis type B and non-A non-B, pyrogenic reactions, and dialysis dementia, to types of infection control practices and strategies, reuse of

Deane, Wineman, and Bemis (eds.): GUIDE TO REPROCESSING OF HEMODIALYZERS.
© 1986. Martinus Nijhoff Publishing. All rights reserved.

dialyzers, and types and concentrations of chemical germicides.

The CDC does not recommend for or against the practice of reusing hemodialyzers but rather has concentrated on the surveillance of diseases that might be associated with dialyzer reuse and on the evaluation of the efficacy of disinfection procedures.

Concept of sterilization and disinfection

The terms *sterilization* and *disinfection* oftentimes are incorrectly used. This is especially true in the dialysis community. The following are classic definitions used in the field of microbiology, and each will be discussed as it is applied in the area of dialysis as well as in the context of reprocessing dialyzers.

Sterilization

Sterilization is a procedure that results in the total destruction of microorganisms including highly resistant bacterial spores. Classically, this is a categorical definition meaning that items that have been subjected to a sterilization process are either sterile or not sterile. From an operational standpoint, however, sterility is defined as the result of a process where the probability of a microorganism surviving on an item subjected to sterilization is less than one chance in a million or 10^{-6}. For example, sterilization processes used by manufacturers of medical devices such as disposable hemodialyzers, involve systems that include the use of good manufacturing practices, validation of the sterilization cycle, use of sophisticated quality control and quality assurance principles, and the application of biologic indicators. In addition, a certain number of items in the sterilized lot are assayed, i.e., sterility tests.

In designing a sterilization process, it is common to assume that the challenge population of microorganisms or the so-called bioburden consists of a large number of bacterial spores. This is a very conservative rationale for designing specific sterilization processes. One should not confuse this sophisticated procedure of quality control and sterilization validation used in the medical device industry with ones that are used in dialysis centers to process and disinfect hemodialyzers. There is virtually no comparison. In the latter instance there is evidence that, if the processing is done correctly by an established protocol, the end result is a reprocessed hemodialyzer that does not appear to have a harmful affect on the patient. As will be pointed out later, however, the process itself is one of disinfection rather than sterilization.

Disinfection

Disinfection is defined as a process that is generally less lethal than sterilization and results in the elimination of most recognized microbial pathogens, not necessarily the more resistant microorganisms that include bacterial endospores. Processes of disinfection can be divided, based on activity, into three broad areas: high-level, intermediate, and low-level disinfection. For purposes of this monograph, only high-level and low-level disinfection will be discussed. (Readers are referred elsewhere for detailed consideration of this concept [2].)

High-level disinfection is a process that inactivates all microorganisms except bacterial spores. For the most part, chemical germicides that are used as high-level disinfectants are capable of inactivating large numbers of bacterial spores after relatively long periods of exposure and consequently are often used as "cold sterilants." When these chemical germicides are used as disinfectants, the exposure period is much shorter (usually 10−30 min at room temperature), which ideally results in all vegetative microorganisms, but not high numbers of bacterial endospores, being inactivated.

Low-level disinfection is a process where many, but not all, microorganisms are inactivated. Low-level disinfection is a means of reducing the microbial population to a level that is considered relatively safe and is virtually synonymous with the term *sanitization*.

In dialysis centers, the fluid pathways of dialysis systems generally are disinfected with chemical germicides such as 1.5% formaldehyde or 200−500 ppm sodium hypochlorite derived from household bleach. The purpose of these procedures is to reduce the microbial population to a safe level in order to prevent septicemia and pyrogenic reactions [3]. Although colloquially the term "sterilization" is used quite often in hemodialysis centers to describe this procedure, it is actually one of disinfection and, more specifically, low-level disinfection.

On the other hand, the use of 2%−4% formaldehyde or other chemical germicides during reprocessing of hemodialyzers for reuse is a procedure that may be high- or low-level disinfection, depending upon the concentration of germicide employed and the contact time, as well as the nature of the microbiologic challenge to which the dialyzer is exposed prior to the disinfection procedure. Normally, the challenge of microorganisms, which will be discussed below, consists of gram-negative water bacteria and, in many cases, nontuberculous mycobacteria.

If a chemical germicide is used in sufficient concentration and contact time, the dialyzer, after the disinfection procedure, may contain no living microorganisms and, in point of fact, be "sterile." However, there is no realistic procedure that a dialysis center can use to verify this state of sterility of individual reprocessed dialyzers. Sophisticated sterility tests require specialized equipment and highly trained microbiologists. Such tests generally cannot be performed in dialysis centers. In fact, none of the assurances that are used by manufacturers of medical devices in labeling disposable dialyzers sterile can be used in a dialysis center. At best, for quality control purposes, a dialysis center can adhere rigidly to established protocols.

MICROBIOLOGIC GUIDELINES FOR WATER

Water for dialysis fluids

Microbiologic guidelines recommended for water and dialysis fluid are based on a number of studies that show that certain types of bacteria, especially the so-called gram-negative water bacteria, can grown rapidly in all types of water prepared for use in dialysis centers. These microorganisms can grow to levels of 10^3-10^6/ml in water prepared by deionization, reverse osmosis, ion exchange, carbon filtration, or distillation. Types of organisms involved would include *Pseudomonas, Alcaligenes, Flavobacterium, Acinetobacter, Serratia,* and *Aeromonas,* to name a few.

Gram-negative microorganisms contain lipopolysaccharide or bacterial endotoxin that can cause pyrogenic reactions in dialyzing patients if the endotoxins are able to enter the vascular system. Water that is produced in a dialysis center for preparing dialysis fluids is not sterile and contains gram-negative water bacteria as well as other types of bacteria. As this water is mixed with dialysate concentrate to produce dialysis fluid, the growth potential of this fluid becomes even greater. As the result of a number of outbreak investigations as well as growth potential studies, two microbiologic guidelines have been recommended.

The first guideline is targeted to water used to prepare dialysis fluid and is based on an estimated degree of amplification of a bacterial population in water as it travels through distribution systems and the artificial kidney machines where it is mixed with dialysis concentrate to produce an isotonic dialysis fluid. It is recommended that the level of microorganisms in water used to prepare dialysis fluid not exceed 200/ml [3, 4].

On the other hand, the microbiologic guidelines for dialysis fluid are based on epidemiologic data showing that high levels of gram-negative bacteria are associated with the risk of pyrogenic reactions in patients who are being dialyzed. It is recommended that the level of microbial contamination in dialysis fluid not exceed 2000/ml [3, 4].

The CDC's surveillance of dialysis-associated diseases, undertaken in collaboration with the HCFA, indicates that currently 99% of chronic dialysis centers in the United States routinely conduct microbiologic assays of water used to prepare dialysis fluid and of dialysis fluid. These tests represent important parts of infection control practices are well as disinfection and sterilization strategy of a dialysis unit. Results of these assays are used to assess the efficacy of disinfection procedures of water treatment systems, and the water and dialysate delivery systems, associated with the artificial kidney machines.

Microbiologic quality of water used in reprocessing hemodialyzers

The disinfection strategy as well as the accompanying microbiologic guidelines for preparing water used to rinse hemodialyzers and to make up solutions of chemical germicides used in the disinfection process differ significantly from those described above (which are targeted to water used to prepare dialysis fluid). Dialysis centers often use "dialysis" grade water to prepare chemical germicides as well as to rinse dialyzers. During the latter two procedures, the dialyzer's microbiologic safety may be compromised. Here especially the microbiologic challenges of these waters are important in the design of a disinfection or sterilization procedure. If the bacteriologic load in water is high, bacteria as well as the accompanying bacterial endotoxins can contaminate the dialyzer and its membranes. Although the microorganisms may be inactivated after treatment with a chemical germicide such as formaldehyde, bacterial endotoxins can remain. Consequently, the sterilization and disinfection strategies for a reuse program in a dialysis center are quite different from those targeted to the water used to prepare dialysis fluid.

Historically, most individuals believed that microbiologic guidelines targeted to water used to prepare dialysis fluid were adequate for water used for rinsing and disinfecting dialyzers. This rationale was based on the assumption that the primary microbiologic challenge in water was composed of gram-negative water bacteria, and the experience that formaldehyde in concentrations of 2% with contact times between 24 and 36 hours appeared to inactivate that particular microbiologic challenge. In 1982, however, at the "National Workshop on Reuse of Consumables on Hemodialysis" held in Washington, DC N.J. Petersen from the CDC [5] pointed out that there is another group of microorganisms that could theoretically cause problems in dialyzer reuse programs. These organisms are the nontuberculous mycobacteria, which are acid-fast water bacteria and, like the gram-negative water bacteria, survive and are capable of rapid growth in all types of water. They do not contain lipopolysaccharide, and their presence in dialysis fluids would tend not to pose a serious risk to a dialyzing patient. Unlike the gram-negative water bacteria, however, they are significantly resistant to chemical germicides [6]. For example, they are $10-100$ times more resistant to free chlorine than *Pseudomonas aeruginosa* and other common gram-negative water bacteria. Some strains of nontuberculous mycobacteria studied at the CDC can survive 60 min of exposure to 2% alkaline gluteraldehyde at room temperature. By comparison, *P. aeruginosa* at a challenge concentration of 10^6 cells/ml would be inactivated within a matter of minutes at room temperature. Some strains of nontuberculous mycobacteria have survived up to 6 h of exposure to 8% formaldehyde at room temperature. In these tests, if the challenge had been *P. aeruginosa*, the inactivation rate would have been so rapid that it could not have been measured. These studies were disturbing because they showed that 2% formaldehyde might not be sufficient to perform high-level disinfection if the primary challenge of microorganisms was nontuberculous mycobacteria. At the meeting in Washington, DC, in 1982, dialysis centers were warned of the possibility of this type of situation. At that time, however, we were not aware of any problems in dialysis centers due to infections caused by these organisms in association with dialyzer reuse programs.

In August of 1982, the CDC received reports of outbreaks of infection caused by *Mycobacterium chelonei* ssp. *abscessus* in two Louisiana hemodialysis centers. Subsequently, a team of epidemiologists and microbiologists investigated these epidemics. A total of 27 cases of nontuberculous mycobacterial infections were identified among 140 patients with end-stage renal disease who had been receiving hemodialysis in the two centers [7].

The results of this epidemiologic investigation indicated that the source of the nontuberculous mycobacteria was water used to rinse dialyzers and to prepare 2% formaldehyde solutions used to disinfect and "pack" hemodialyzers for storage until their next use. Nontuberculous mycobacteria were detected in the blood compartments of five of 31 dialyzers sampled after routine disinfection procedures with 2% formaldehyde. Although there was evidence that a concentration of 2% formaldehyde was not always reached in some dialyzers, subsequent laboratory studies showed that the nontuberculous mycobacteria associated with the particular water system in the two centers could readily survive 2% formaldehyde after 24 h of exposure at room temperature. Some strains of nontuberculous mycobacteria can survive up to 96 h of exposure to 2% formaldehyde [8].

In one study, a strain of nontuberculous mycobacteria isolated from the dialysis center involved in the outbreak of infections mentioned above was exposed to 2% formaldehyde within a hemodialyzer as well as in laboratory test tube conditions. Results summarized in table 4-1 indicate similar findings in both types of test systems. A 1.7-log reduction of the nontuberculous mycobacteria occurred within 24 h, but after four days of exposure, 65 viable organisms/ml still remained.

Further studies showed that, if the concentration of formaldehyde is increased to 4%, none of the strains of nontuberculous mycobacteria associated with the outbreak in Louisiana, which have been considered the most resistant strains of nontuberculous mycobacteria, survived beyond 24 h of exposure at room temperature.

At this point it appeared to us that the use of 2% formaldehyde as a procedure for disinfection of disposable hemodialyzers was marginal at best. Perhaps if the microbiologic challenge consisted of gram-negative water bacteria, the reprocessed dialyzer could be interpreted as being safe to use. Even this would be debatable because the artificial kidney is considered a critical medical device that is exposed to the vascular system and that should be subjected to a true sterilization process. On the other hand, if nontuberculous mycobacteria comprised the microbiologic challenge, the use of 2% formaldehyde would have to be considered inadequate. In 1983, it was recommended that, if formaldehyde were used as the chemical germicide to reprocess hemodialyzers, its concentration should be at least 4% [9].

In 1984, the CDC conducted a survey to determine the prevalence of

Table 4-1. Resistance of nontuberculous mycobacteria to 2% formaldehyde at room temperature (22°C−25°C)

Inocula/ ml[2]	Test condition	Length of exposure	Mean results (cfu/ml)	Log reduction
6.3×10^5	Dialyzer	24 h	1.1×10^4	1.8
6.3×10^5	Test tube	24 h	1.4×10^4	1.7
1.2×10^6	Dialyzer	48 h	2.7×10^1	4.7
5.0×10^5	Test tube	72 h	9.5×10^0	4.7
1.2×10^6	Dialyzer	96 h	6.5×10^1	4.3

[2]Inocula used as diluent to prepare 2% formaldehyde.

nontuberculous mycobacteria in water used in chronic hemodialysis centers. Dialysis centers invited to participate in the study were chosen at random from 1171 centers in the national listing of providers furnishing kidney dialysis and transplant services [10]. Water samples were collected from 115 dialysis centers over a 13-week study period. In general, the results of this survey, which are not yet published, showed that nontuberculous mycobacteria were present in the water of 83% of the dialysis centers surveyed. Thus nontuberculous mycobacteria can be considered to be part of the normal microbial flora in water and the microbiologic challenge when designing disinfection and sterilization procedures. These findings reinforce the recommendation to use 4% Formaldehyde or equivalent germicides rather than 2% formaldehyde when disinfecting dialyzers.

The question often arises: If the microbiologic quality of water used to prepare dialysis fluid meets the CDC and AAMI guidelines, can this water be safely used in reprocessing programs, i.e., to rinse dialyzers and to prepare chemical germicides? Not necessarily. As mentioned above, the microbiologic guidelines targeted to water used to prepare dialysis fluid are designed to control gram-negative water bacteria and to prevent pyrogenic reactions and septicemia. Disinfection strategies that result in relatively low numbers of bacteria, as determined by assays with culture plates (incubated for no longer than 48 h), might reasonably be considered indicative of relatively good quality water. This is not guaranteed, however, because the standard microbiologic assays for water used to prepare dialysis fluid do not indicate the number of nontuberculous mycobacteria present. A 48-h incubation time is too short for colonies of nontuberculous mycobacteria to develop and, more importantly, there are no data to suggest the level of nontuberculous mycobacteria that constitutes a risk of the organism surviving the disinfection procedure. Further, the techniques involved in detecting and enumerating nontuberculous mycobacteria are complex and could not be performed in a routine fashion in dialysis centers.

The dialysis center then is faced with two alternatives for dealing with nontuberculous mycobacteria as a challenge to the disinfection procedure of reused dialyzers. On the one hand, one could use completely aseptic techniques throughout the reprocessing procedure, use sterile rinse water and sterile disinfectant (probably membrane filter sterilized), and employ strict quality control. In our opinion, most centers are not capable of operating a closed-system approach. The second option would be to use a chemical germicide having the bactericidal activity capability of 4% formaldehyde. Although good quality control, quality assurance, and adherence to protocols would have to be maintained, this is the simpler alternative. In addition, there is scientific information indicating that 4% formaldehyde for 24 h of exposure at room temperature is at least a high-level disinfection, if not a sterilization process. All laboratory data acquired so far show that 24 h of exposure to 4% formaldehyde at room temperature inactivates large numbers of all strains of nontuberculous bacteria tested. Many of the test strains are among the most resistant in our collection.

It should be emphasized that both the dialysate and blood compartments of each dialyzer must be filled with 4% formaldehyde to prevent a reduction in the concentration due to diffusion of formaldehyde from one compartment to the other. Also, residual rinse water contained on and in the dialyzer fibers will dilute the chemical germicide to some lesser concentration unless at least 3 compartment-volumes of formaldehyde are passed through each compartment before the dialyzer is sealed for storage.

In summary, there are no specific microbiologic guidelines for water used to rinse reprocessed hemodialyzers or to prepare chemical germicides. Reliance is made upon the use of chemical germicides at sufficient concentrations to inactivate large numbers of nontuberculous mycobacteria.

CHEMICAL GERMICIDES OTHER THAN FORMALDEHYDE

In recent years, several manufacturers have formulated a number of chemical germicides to disinfect and, in most cases, to sterilize reprocessed hemodialyzers. These germicides include the active ingredients of alkaline glutaraldehyde, glutaraldehyde and phenate, peracetic acid and hydrogen peroxide, chlorine dioxide, and organic hypochlorous acid complex. A number of investigators are conducting studies to evaluate these chemical germicides. Results presented at a recent meeting on the reuse of hemodialyzers (sponsored by the AAMI, Los Angeles, 5–6 November 1984) indicated that virtually all of these newer germicides were equivalent or superior in bactericidal activity to 4% formaldehyde. (See chapter 2 for other information.)

As mentioned elsewhere in this monograph, the bactericidal efficiency of the chemical germicide is only one factor used in judging it suitability for disinfecting hemodialyzers. An equally important factor is the ability of the reprocessing protocol to rinse the chemical germicide from the hemodialyzer. It is possible that a chemical germicide might be very effective as a bactericide, but not be efficiently rinsed from a dialyzer. Germicides also are potentially capable of damaging the membranes of the dialyzer. Such agents would not be useful in a dialyzer-reuse program.

BACTERIAL ENDOTOXIN

Pyrogenic reactions attributed to bacterial endotoxins are a common risk associated with hemodialysis [11]. Although the CDC−HCFA surveillance of dialysis-associated diseases between 1976 and 1983 did not indicate an association between reuse of hemodialyzers and increased risk of pyrogenic reactions, the CDC routinely receives requests for assistance in investigating pyrogenic reactions from dialysis centers practicing reuse of dialyzers. Many investigations disclosed that sporadic pyrogenic reactions occurred in patients dialyzed with reused dialyzers, but not in patients using new dialyzers. In each instance, the aqueous formaldehyde solution used to disinfect the dialyzers before reuse was prepared either with water that had not been treated to remove endotoxins or with treated water that had been allowed to stand in a tank for several days before use, thus permitting growth of gram-negative water bacteria and production of large amounts of endotoxins. Under both of these circumstances, levels of endotoxin capable of causing pyrogenic reactions were detected in the water used to prepare the disinfectant solution [5].

Migration of the endotoxin from the disinfectant solution to the dialyzer's membranes or the membrane potting material has been shown to occur when the dialyzer, after reprocessing with a disinfectant solution containing endotoxin, is stored for 1−2 days. Removal of this endotoxin material will not be complete when the disinfectant is rinsed from the dialyzer prior to reuse [12]. The amount of endotoxin retained by a dialyzer during disinfection seems to vary. Factors affecting its retention are the concentration of endotoxin in the disinfectant, the type of dialyzer or dialyzer membrane material, plus some as yet unknown factor related to previous use of the dialyzer. We have not noticed significant retention of endotoxin material by the dialyzer when only the rinse water was contaminated with endotoxin.

To prevent pyrogenic reactions (from this source of endotoxin), the water used to prepare disinfectant solutions should not contain appreciable amounts of endotoxin. We have not seen pyrogenic reactions associated with disinfectant solutions containing endotoxin at levels less than 1 ng/ml. Consequently we suggest that a reasonable maximum endotoxin level for water used to prepare the disinfectant would be 1 ng/ml.

CHEMICALS

Maximum levels for chemical contaminants in the water used to prepare dialysate were established by the AAMI in 1982 because of concern for the recognized risks and hazards to hemodialysis patients. At the time of development of this AAMI standard it was not possible to address all potentially harmful contaminants because of the lack of reliable information on their health effects, especially in the area of hemodialysis. Special concern continues to be expressed about the exposure of hemodialysis patients to such contaminants as organic chemicals and various trace metals. The risk posed by these contaminants, especially the metals, to dialysis patients is exacerbated by their longer biologic retention times in hemodialysis patients, resulting from absent or compromised urinary excretion. Continued accumulation of the contaminating trace metals in various body tissues of patients can be expected, with consequent development of potential problems. Dialysis encephalopathy caused by cumulative aluminum exposure via dialysate is an example of such an exposure to a metal contaminant [13]. It is not known whether additional exposure to such a contaminant may result from reuse of a hemodialyzer that has been rinsed in potable water, stored in a disinfectant prepared with potable water, and then rinsed with 500−1000 ml of sterile, pyrogen-free saline. The potential risks and hazards to the hemodialysis patient specifically associated with organic chemical contaminants in water are also unknown.

There is still concern, however, with the chemical quality of municipal water supplied to the dialysis center. In a recent publication by the Environmental Protection Agency (EPA) on volatile synthetic organic chemicals, it was pointed out that 99 (21.2%) of 466 randomly selected groundwater supplies had at least one volatile organic chemical contaminant [14]. Typically, contamination was at low levels, but a few samples had high levels of some of the contaminants. Even in situations in which specific contaminants have been identified, there is no consensus on what constitutes a safe, acceptable level of contamination for potable water supplies, let alone for any specialized areas of water usage such as for hemodialysis. Some feel that safe levels of volative organic chemicals cannot be determined from available health-effects data. Similar controversy exists for other organic chemical groups such as chlorinated hydrocarbons and trihalomethanes.

Dialysis centers are advised to take a conservative approach in their selection of the chemical quality requirements for water to be used in dialyzer reprocessing programs. It may be prudent to treat at least the water used to prepare the dialyzer disinfectant in a manner that would substantially remove potential chemical contaminants.

REFERENCES

1. Alter MJ, Favero MS, Petersen NJ, Doto IL, Leger RT, Maynard JE: National surveillance of dialysis-associated hepatitis and other diseases 1976 and 1980. Dial Transplant 12:860−868, 1983.
2. Favero MS: Chemical disinfection of medical and surgical materials. In: Block SS (ed Disinfection, sterilization and preservation, 3rd edn. Lea and Febiger, Philadelphia, 1983, pp 469−492.
3. Favero MS, Petersen NJ: Microbiological guidelines for hemodialysis systems. Dial Transplant 6:34−36, 1977.
4. Association for the Advencement of Medical Instrumentation: American national standard for hemodialysis systems. Association for the Advancement of Medical Instrumentation, Arlington VA, 1981.

5. Petersen NJ: Microbiologic hazards associated with reuse of hemodialyzers. In: Proceedings of national workshop on reuse of consumables in hemodialysis. Kidney Disease Coalition, Baltimore, 1982, pp 121–129.
6. Carson LA, Petersen NJ, Favero MS, Aguero SM: Growth characteristics of atypical mycobacteria in water and their comparative resistance to disinfectants. Appl Environ Microbiol 36:839–846, 1978.
7. Bolan G.A,. Reingold AL, Carson LA, et al.: Infections with *Mycobacterium chelonei* in patients receiving dialysis and using processed hemodialyzers. J. Infect. Dis. 152: 1013–1019, 1985.
8. Bland LA, Alter MJ, Favero MS, Carson LA, Cusick LB: Hemodialyzer reuse: practices in the United States and implication for infection control. Trans Am Soc Artif Intern Organs 31: 556–559 1985.
9. Favero MS: Distinguishing between high-level disinfection, reprocessing, and sterilization. AAMI Technology Assessment Report no. 6–83. Association for the Advancement of Medical Instrumentation, Arlington VA, 1983.
10. Health Care Financing Administration: National listing of providers furnishing kidney dialysis and transplant services. Baltimore, 1983.
11. Food and Drug Administration Medical Device Standards Publication Technical Report: Investigation of the risks and hazards associated with hemodialysis devices. Contract 223-78-5046, April 1980.
12. Petersen NJ, Carson LA, Favero MS: Bacterial endotoxin in new and reused hemodialyzers: a potential cause of endotoxemia. Trans Am Soc Artif Intern Organs 27:155–160, 1981.
13. Schreeder MT, Favero MS, Hughes JR, Petersen NJ, et al.: Dialysis encephalopathy and aluminum exposure: an epidemiologic analysis. J Chronic Dis 36:581–593, 1983.
14. Environmental Protection Agency: National primary drinking water regulations: volatile synthetic organic chemicals; proposed rulemaking. Fed Register 49: 24330–24355, 1984.

5. RECORD-KEEPING PROCEDURES FOR DIALYZER REUSE

NATHAN W. LEVIN
ANTHONY MESSANA
MARY ANN MILLER-MESSANA

The subject of quality control is covered in some of its dimensions by other contributors to this volume (see chapter 12). Documentation or record keeping is hardly the most dramatic subject to discuss, but it is an essential ingredient in quality control.

Until recently, the reuse of dialyzers was largely a manual procedure, and the variability in quality control and in documentation was obvious. In many instances, quality control was virtually nonexistent except for the measurements of fiber bundle volume. Record keeping for the most part was poor and inconsistent.

The use of automated procedures has encouraged better record keeping, largely because the records are easier to maintain. In addition, now that reuse techniques are more widely used, legal pressures are increasing. The recommendations or projected guidelines of organizations, such as the Association for Advancement of Medical Instrumentation or the National Kidney Foundation, definitely affect those who are thinking about dialyzer reprocessing.

QUALITY CONTROL

Quality control starts before the reprocessing procedure actually begins with documentation of the materials to be used. The dialyzers must be in good condition without cracks or leaks, the equipment for testing must be validated, and written protocols for all aspects of the reprocessing procedure must be available for everyone in the unit and for outside agencies empo-

Deane, Wineman, and Bemis (eds.) GUIDE TO REPROCESSING OF HEMODIALYZERS.
© 1986. Martinus Nijhoff Publishing. All rights reserved.

wered to inspect such protocols.

Written protocols should address the following: (1) training and retraining of technicians, indicating that those who perform the procedures are qualified; (2) methods of cleaning; (3) disinfectant detection, both in the fluids used for reuse and in the environment; (4) patient and staff safety techniques in use in the unit; (5) detection of endotoxin pyrogens in the water used for reuse; and (6) water treatment, e.g., a bacterial culture of bacteria and chemical content of reverse osmosis water. Detailed descriptions of all reprocessing methods, whether automated or manual, are essential.

Quality control must also inlcude consideration of patient complaints; not merely the complaints about the reprocessing techniques themselves, but also the complaints about first-use versus reuse symptoms. By effective reprocessing, it is possible to restore biocompatibility to its initial level, which could be undesirable. In at least one automated system where bleach is used during reprocessing, the biochemical situation produced by the new dialyzer is created, i.e., complement activation. However, it appears that clinical symptoms may be ameliorated despite this. Before the initiation of hemodialysis in a facility utilizing dialyzer reprocessing, each patient should be educated as to the reuse procedure as well as the related risks and advantages. Documentation of signed informed consent to dialyzer reuse should be present on the patient's chart.

Two final requirements of quality control are the need to perform audits and to educate patients, their families, and often the media. The audits are a device by which the quality control is verified by checking that forms, policies, and procedures are being followed. The issue of dialyzer reuse has received a great deal of public attention.

It is necessary to evaluate the quality control in the reprocessing of the hemodialyzer itself. There are currently several different types of disinfectants being used. Formaldehyde is most commonly used, though not without risks and hazards to both patients and staff. Other products, such as glutaraldehydes and peracetic acid are being evaluated and hold some hope for a less hazardous disinfectant (see chapter 2). Documentation in the form of checking for the presence of a disinfectant prior to patient use as well as the lowering of the disinfectant level to acceptable limits just prior to the initiation of dialysis is required. The presence of disinfectant may be determined through the addition of dye, measurement of the viscosity, or commercially available reagents.

A word is necessary concerning the potential hazards of disinfectants, especially formaldehyde. Proper awareness in the form of staff and patient education and policies is necessary. This is especially important due to the recently recommended practice of increasing the percentage of formaldehyde to 4%. Documentation must include the monitoring of formaldehyde air levels and the reporting of any formaldehyde accidents. Disinfectant spills should be cleaned up using proper procedures as determined by the unit.

Table 5-1. List of suggested forms[2] for reprocessing and quality assurance

Reprocessing forms	Quality assurance forms
Form 1 Dialyzer label	Form 8 Dialyzer priming volumes
Form 2 Dialy reuse log	Form 9 Dailyzer BUN clearances
Form 3 Discard list	Form 10 Water iodine level report
Form 4 Individual patient reprocessing Report	Form 11 Endotoxin level report
Form 5 Dialyzer usage monthly report	Form 12 Bacteriological results
Form 6 Dialyzer reuse program summary	Form 13 Dialyzer bacteriological results
Form 7 Reuse activity calendar	Form 14 Possible pyrogenic reaction
	Form 15 Formaldehyde air sampling
	Form 16 Formaldehyde incident report

[a] The forms, as illustrated in the accompanying figures, are suggested for recording and documentation, and serve only as examples of those appropriate for legal and scientific purposes. The forms are copyright by Fairlane Health Services Corporation, Dearborn, Michigan, and should not be reproduced without permission of this organization.

DOCUMENTATION

In any reprocessing program, the framework for documentation of each step of all procedures must be present. The following are examples of such a program. With direct documentation, it should be possible to follow a patient's dialyzer from its first use until it fails to pass prescribed tests and is discarded. All quality assurance steps should be documented. Thus both the framework and detailed entries should be currently maintained.

Dialyzer labeling (figure 5-1)

This provides the important first step in any reprocessing procedure, whether manual or automated. The label contains the following information: patient name, total blood volume, reuse number, date and time disinfected, and the release date and time. A new label should be on the dialyzer for the first use and for each subsequent use.

For the manual system, the total blood compartment volume is compared with the reference volume for that type of dialyzer. Each dialysis unit establishes the percentage of reference volume acceptable for a dialyzer to be reused.

In the automated systems, the reprocessing machine checks the kidney according to dialyzer type and performs various tests to insure the integrity of the dialyzer for continued treatments.

The dialyzers are stored containing appropriate disinfectant and are not to be used until sufficient time has elapsed, in accordance with current standards.

In this system, the reuse number is the total number of times the dialyzer has been reprocessed. New dialyzers have a reuse value of zero, after the first reprocessing the reuse number becomes 1.

NAME _____

VOLUME _____

REUSE _____

| RELEASE DATE _____ |
| RELEASE TIME _____ |

DATE DISINFECTED _____

TIME DISINFECTED _____

DO NOT USE UNTIL AFTER RELEASE DATE AND TIME.
© 1982 Fairlane Health Services Corporation L- 83

Figure 5-1. The dialyzer label.

Fairlane Health Services
DAILY REUSE LOG

DATE: _____   SHIFT _____

PATIENT NAME	DIALYZER INFO				DISCARD INFORMATION					SIGNATURE
	TYPE	REF. VOL.	USE #	RES. VOL.	DISCARD LIST	LOW RES. VOLUME	BLOOD LEAK	HEADER LEAK	OTHER*	

*EXPLAIN ALL "OTHERS": _____

Figure 5-2. The daily reuse log.

Daily reuse log (figures 5-2 and 5-3)

This log sheet is an overview of the day's total reuse activity. Each dialyzer is recorded by patient's name, dialyzer type, reuse number, reference (original) blood volume, and residual blood volume. If residual volume falls below the determined cutoff percentage of the reference volume, that dialyzer will be discarded. Other common reasons for discard are listed. A *discard list* contains the names of all patients who, by facility policy, do not use reprocessed dialyzers (see figure 5-4).

Fairlane Health Services
DISCARD LIST

NAME	DATE	REASON

Figure 5-3. The discard list.

Fairlane Health Services
INDIVIDUAL REPROCESSING REPORT

PATIENT NAME _____ MONTH_____

DATE	DIALYZER INFORMATION				DISCARD INFORMATION					SIGNATURE
	TYPE	REF. VOL.	USE #	RES. VOL.	DISCARD LIST	LOW RES. VOLUME	BLOOD LEAK	HEADER LEAK	OTHER*	

TOTALS	DIALYZER TYPES	NEW	TXS	DISCARD LIST	LOW RES. VOL.	BLOOD LEAK	HEADER LEAK	OTHER*

Figure 5-4. The individual reprocessing report.

Reasons for discard other than those given on this form are indicated under *other* and explained briefly at the bottom of the page.

Individual patient documentation (figure 5-4)

With this log, the reuse activity for one patient's dialyzer(s) can be recorded. Using this information, problems such as underheparinization, poor access, and poor recirculation may be reflected in poor reuse numbers, and can be addressed.

The information is transferred from the daily reuse log to the individual reprocessing report. The information is recorded under the same columns that are utilized for the daily reuse log. At the end of the month, the experience of each dialyzer type is totaled and the appropriate information is inserted at the bottom of each form.

A different form is used to record the patients' dialyzers on a monthly basis for the automated system. The automated machine generates a set of two (2) labels, one to be placed on the dialyzer, and one on this form. The technician initials this documentation. The information is totaled at the bottom of each sheet.

Dialyzer usage: monthly report (figure 5-5)

This listing is utilized to analyze the experience of each dialyzer type during that month. Listed are the names of each patient utilizing that dialyzer type,

DIALYZER USAGE: MONTHLY REPORT							
DIALYZER TYPE				MONTH			
PATIENT NAME	USES	NEW	AVERAGE	PATIENT NAME	USES	NEW	AVERAGE

	USES	NEW	AVERAGE
TOTAL			

Figure 5-5. The monthly report of dialyzer usage.

DIALYZER REUSE PROGRAM SUMMARY

MONTH OF ——————, 198—

DIALYZER TYPE	TXS	– – – –TOTAL REUSE – – – –NEW DIALYZERS	REUSE AVERAGE	TXS	– – – W/O DISCARDS – – – –NEW DIALYZERS	REUSE AVERAGE

TOTALS

DISCARD SUMMARY

DIALYZER TYPE	LOW VOLUME	BLOOD LEAK	CLOTTED DIALYZER	DISCARD LIST	OTHER

TOTALS

Figure 5-6. The dialyzer reuse program summary.

the number of uses, or "treatments", received by each patient for each type of dialyzer and the number of new dialyzers used for each patient. These numbers are compiled from the *individual reprocessing report* (figure 5-3). From these numbers, the average number of uses per dialyzer per patient can be caluclated and entered. At the page bottom are the overall reuse statistics for each dialyzer type.

REUSE ACTIVITY CALENDAR 1984

GHSC — TOLEDO
OVERALL REUSE

(WITH DISCARDS)

	JAN	FEB	MAR	APR	MAY	JUN	JUL	AUG	SEP	OCT	NOV	DEC	Y-T-D
TOTAL TXS	383	439	604	477	457	572	484	506	489	645	409	626	6091
DIALYZERS	122	137	153	102	91	108	78	95	106	159	97	156	1404
REUSE AVE	3.1	3.2	3.9	4.7	5.0	5.3	6.2	5.3	4.3	4.1	4.2	4.0	4.3

DIALYZER SPECIFIC

(WITHOUT DISCARDS)

		JAN	FEB	MAR	APR	MAY	JUN	JUL	AUG	SEP	OCT	NOV	DEC	T-T-D
A	TREATMENT	70	126	186	130	127	162	156	149	118	171	0	132	1527
	DIALYZERS	24	35	26	15	18	28	13	23	19	21	0	20	242
	AVE REUSE	2.9	3.6	7.2	8.7	7.1	5.8	12.0	6.5	6.2	8.1	ERR	6.6	6.3
B	TREATMENT	267	267	317	268	264	350	288	322	322	358	347	392	3762
	DIALYZERS	57	62	36	20	25	33	30	43	45	34	51	53	489
	AVE REUSE	4.7	4.3	8.8	13.4	10.6	10.6	9.6	7.5	7.2	10.5	6.8	7.4	7.7
C	TREATMENT	12	12	14	15	20	15	6	8	8	16	20	22	168
	DIALYZERS	7	6	4	3	2	2	1	2	1	4	4	3	39
	AVE REUSE	1.7	2.0	3.5	5.0	10.0	7.5	6.0	4.0	8.0	4.0	5.0	7.3	4.3
TOTAL	TREATMENT	349	405	517	413	411	527	450	479	448	545	367	546	5457
	DIALYZERS	88	103	66	38	45	63	44	68	65	59	55	76	770
	AVE REUSE	4.0	4.0	7.8	10.8	9.1	8.4	10.2	7.0	6.9	9.2	6.7	7.2	7.1

Figure 5-7. The reuse activity calendar.

MONTH:_____

"NEW" Dialyzer Priming Volume Measurements

Dialyzer Type	# to Measure	1	2	3	4	5	6	7	8	9	10	mean volume	cutoff volume

Figure 5-8. The "new" dialyzer priming volume measurements.

Dialyzer reuse program summary (figure 5-6)

At the end of each month, a summary is made that provides an overall analysis based on dialyzer types, total treatments on that dialyzer type, and total number of dialyzers used. The average number of uses per dialyzer is calculated with and without discards.

The discard summary records the information based on individual dialyzers. The information is drawn from the individual reprocessing report summary at the bottom of the page. This provides an overview of the program's effectiveness, and compares reusability of dialyzer types and any trends that are developing.

Reuse activity calendar (figure 5-7)

At the end of each month, in a multi-unit program, each individual unit completes the dialyzer reuse program summary. This information is compiled in the reuse activity calendar. This form provides a month-by-month average overall, in addition to being dialyzer specific. Included in this form is a year-to-date column that gives more comprehensive data for the reprocessing program. This form is individualized to each unit based on dialyzer type and method of reuse. If a unit is doing both manual and automated reuse, the information must be analyzed further to give actual data based on automated only, manual only, and combined automated and manual reuse.

This tool illustrates the effectiveness of the dialyzer reprocessing program, giving insight to trends. It also provides information as to the reusability of various types of dialyzers.

"New" dialyzer priming volume measurements (figure 5-8)

This form is utilized in order to establish current primary total blood compartment volume for each dialyzer type used. A percentage of the average number of each type of dialyzer is tested each month, and each initial volume is recorded. The mean volume for each dialyzer type is then calculated. The cutoff volume can then be determined according to facility policy.

Figure 5–9. The dialyzer BUN clearance.

Figure 5-10. The water iodine level report.

Figure 5-11. The endotoxin level report.

Dialyzer BUN clearance (figure 5-9)

On this form is a record of performance of BUN clearance studies and documentation of the dialysis parameters affecting its outcome (QB and TMP). Included is a summary of the recommended study procedure and the formula for actual calculation of BUN clearance.

Water iodine level report (figure 5-10)

This serves as a log of water iodine levels taken throughout the year. Acceptable iodine levels will be specified by dialysis unit policy. Maintaining an established level of iodine provides assurance as to the continued acceptability of the water.

Fairlane Health Services
BACTERIOLOGICAL LEVEL REPORT FORM

DATE	LOCATION	RESULTS	SIGNATURE	DATE	LOCATION	RESULTS	SIGNATURE

Figure 5-12. The bacteriological level report.

Fairlane Health Services
DIALYZER BACTERIOLOGY RESULTS
MONTH _____

DATE	PT. NAME	TYPE	USE	RESULTS	SIGNATURE

Figure 5-13 The dialyzer bacteriology results.

Endotoxin level report (figure 5-11)

In investigating a suspected pyrogenic reaction, a water sample is taken from the outlet at the appropriate patient station and analyzed for endotoxin level. The entries on this form should coincide directly with those of form 14 (figure 5-14).

Bacteriological level report (figure 5-12)

On this log sheet are recorded the results of bacteria colony counts drawn routinely throughout the dialysis unit. Industry standard has long been that colony count in product water should not exceed 200 colonies/ml. Recent Centers for Disease Control advice suggests replacement by limulus amoebocyte lysate (endotoxin) testing. This form should also record mycobacterial test results. No mycobacterial colonies should be present during testing.

Dialyzer bacteriology results (figure 5-13)

Routine cultures on reused dialyzers insure that proper disinfection is taking place. A percentage of dialyzers, new and reused, may be cultured for the presence of bacteria and mycobacteria. The results are recorded on this form and include the following information: date of culture, patient name, dialyzer type, use number, results, and signature of the person recording the results. Dialyzer colony counts should be zero if proper disinfecting procedures are followed. This is one of the procedures to be documented in any system, to show that the reused dialyzers are safe for patient use.

Fairlane Health Services
POSSIBLE PYROGEN REACTION FORM

DATE	PATIENT NAME	DIALYZER		BODY TEMPERATURE		CHILLS/ FEVER?
		TYPE	USE	PRE	POST	

Figure 5-14. Possible pyrogenic reaction.

Fairlane Health Services
FORMALDEHYDE AIR SAMPLING

DATE	TIME	RESULTS

Figure 5-15. Formaldehyde air sampling.

Fairlane Health Services
FORMALDEHYDE INCIDENT REPORT FORM

Date of incident _____ Employee Name _____

Area where incident occurred _____

Description of incident:

Signature of Supervisor _____

Signature of Head Nurse _____

Signature of Employee _____

Was Physician Notified ? Yes _____ No _____

Description of Actions taken

Figure 5-16. The formadehyde incident report.

Possible pyrogenic reaction (figure 5-14)

The information recorded is very basic, limited to date and patient name, dialyzer type, and use number. Documentation of physical symptoms includes only pre- and posttreatment body temperature and whether chills and fever were present. More detailed medical information is present in the patient chart.

Formaldehyde air sampling (figure 5-15)

It is necessary to limit the exposure of employees to formaldehyde. This sampling insures that appropriate techniques are employed to limit the exposure. This form provides documentation as to the level of formaldehyde encountered by employees in the workplace. Information on this form includes the date the test was performed, the duration of sampling, and the results. This record should be kept for future reference. The form can be used as an indicator of whether employees are following proper procedures, and also can reflect adequacy of ventilation in dialyzer reprocessing areas.

Formaldehyde Incident Report (figure 5-16)

This form provides the necessary documentation in the event of an employee's exposure to an excessive amount of formaldehyde. This form is used in such instances as a large formaldehyde spill or where the employee gets splashed with formaldehyde. Signatures of the employee, head nurse, and supervisor are necessary in addition to a description of the incident and actions taken. Physician notification and his recommendations are to be included.

6. CLINICAL RESPONSES TO NEW AND REPROCESSED HEMODIALYZERS

DAVID A. OGDEN

Hemodialysis has always been and continues to be associated with adverse symptoms as well as benefits. The dialysis disequilibrium syndrome, including headache, lassitude, occasional convulsions, nausea, vomiting, muscle cramps, and hypotension, was described more than 20 years ago [1, 2], and today remains to some degree a problem with every dialysis. This syndrome is a consequence of achieving zero balance dialysis, particularly of sodium chloride, water, urea, and total osmoles, using intermittent therapy.

The history of hemodialysis is replete with reports of toxicity of materials used in dialysis and of medications used by dialysis patients [3]. Dialysis membranes, polyvinylchloride (PVC) tubing, sterilizing agents, disinfecting agents, machines and plumbing, water, concentrate, heparin, and intravenous fluids have all been implicated in toxic reactions in dialysis patients. Blood transfusions, iron therapy, aluminum hydroxide, calcium salts, and vitamins also have had adverse effects on dialysis patients.

It is in this setting (where subtle or overt reactions are commonplace) that the clinical responses from new and reprocessed dialyzers must be assessed.

Dialyzer reuse was stimulated by the extremely high cost of the early disposable-coil, parallel-plate, and hollow-fiber dialyzers; the very limited funds available to treat patients with chronic renal failure in the 1960s and early 1970s; and the use of the Kiil dialyzer, which required rebuilding with new membranes and blood ports and formaldehyde disinfection before the next use. During the mid-1970s, dialyzers of all configurations became

Deane, Wineman, and Bemis (eds.): GUIDE TO REPROCESSING OF HEMODIALYZERS.
© 1986. Martinus Nijhoff Publishing. All rights reserved.

available at moderate prices as the number of dialysis patients, and therefore the number of dialyzers needed, increased dramatically, and as funds became available from Medicare payments for dialysis. Reuse was then practiced by only a limited number of facilities. In the late 1970s, increasing costs due to inflation, which were not accompanied by increases in Medicare reimbursement for dialysis, again provided an economic incentive for reuse. At about the same time, it became apparent that new dialyzers were associated with occasionally severe patient reactions [4], and frequent mild to moderate patient reactions [4, 5] (figures 1-1 and 1-2 of chapter 1). Moreover, it was demonstrated that these reactions were greatly reduced during dialysis with previously used and reprocessed dialyzers [5, 6].

The widespread and still growing practice of dialyzer reuse today is, therefore, based on both economic and medical considerations.

SAFETY OF NEW DIALYZERS

Manufacture of new dialyzers is controlled by the Food and Drug Administration's Good Manufacturing Practices (GMP) regulations. A relatively small number of manufacturers (each using somewhat different production techniques) produce new dialyzers. Quality control and quality assurance methods, carefully designed and strictly applied, using process controls and sample validation methods, permit standards of performance (manufacturing specifications) to be achieved. Sterilization of the final product is accomplished with ethylene oxide gas or irradiation.

New dialyzers are not supplied ready for use. They must first be processed by the facility by flushing of the blood compartment with 15−20 vol of sterile normal saline, while simultaneously flushing the dialysate compartment with dialysate. Alternatively, many facilities flush the blood compartment with an initial small rinse of normal saline that is recirculated for 15−25 min while flushing the dialysate compartment with dialysate at 500 ml/min. A final blood compartment flush of 500 ml of normal saline is then performed.

NEW DIALYZER SYNDROME

Failure to perform a copious blood compartment flush has been associated with a striking increase in serious and sometimes fatal patient reactions [7]. Even when processed before use, serious and fatal reactions may occur. Such reactions have been named the *new dialyzer syndrome* [4] or *first-use syndrome* [8]. Reports of such reactions are surely incomplete, yet for the years 1982 and 1983, the Food and Drug Administration received 366 reports of first-use syndrome, 85% of which were classified as severe reactions, and 11 of which were fatal. Accordingly, during those two years, approximately five of every 1000 hemodialysis patients suffered a severe reaction, and approximately one in 10,000 suffered a fatal reaction to a new dialyzer. The vast majority of the dialyzers implicated were CUPROPHAN® hollow-fiber dialyzers [9].

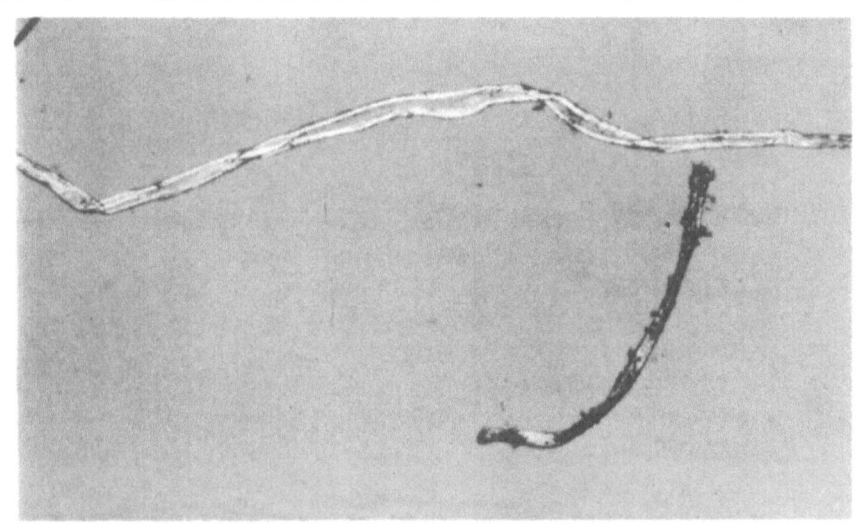

Figure 6-1. Particulates recovered from a hollow-fiber dialyzer. Enlarged 120 times. Actual length approximately 1 mm.

The cause of patient reactions to new dialyzers is not specifically known, although recent work has done much to improve our understanding of patient–dialyzer reactions. It is probable that such reactions are multifactorial, and may be caused either by residua of the manufacturing process, by the membrane itself, or by both.

At this point it is appropriate to point out that clinical observations and clinical studies of patient reactions may fail to differentiate between the dialyzer itself and the arterial and venous blood line sets, usually made of PVC, as a source of either residua of manufacture or of blood–material bioincompatibility since both are necessary for clinical dialysis. Unless specifically noted, therefore, either may be the source of the agent involved in the referenced studies that follow.

PARTICULATES

New dialyzers contain particulates. In a recent study (D.A. Ogden, unpublished), particulates of a variety of sizes and shapes up to 1 mm long were found in the filtered effluent from the blood compartment of both hollow-fiber (figure 6-1) and parallel-plate (figure 6-2) dialyzers. The total weight of particulates in the first and second liter of filtered blood compartment effluent was 1.2–2.2 mg and 0.8–1.1 mg, respectively. No reactions have been attributed to infusion of these particulates into dialysis patients. Some, but clearly not all, would be removed by the dialyzer blood compartment flush before initiating dialysis. However, 1 mg infused with each dialysis would constitute a burden of more than 150 mg a year, or over 1 g in seven years of

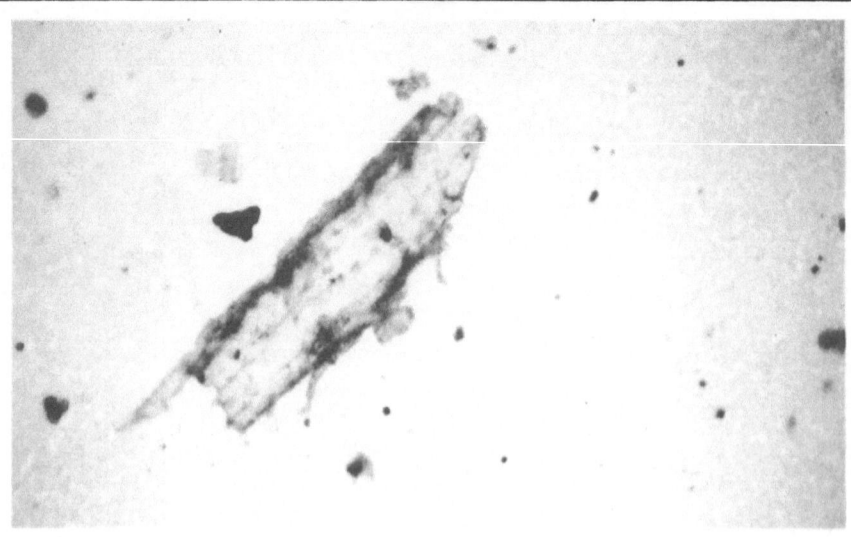

Figure 6-2. Particulates recovered from a parallel-plate dialyzer. Enlarged 120 times. Actual lengthof largest particle approximately 0.5 mm.

dialysis. Intravenous (i.v.) fluids, particularly those packaged in glass containers some years ago, contained particulates capable of causing granulomatous vascular and pulmonary lesions in humans [10]. A study utilizing rabbits infused with standard i.v. solutions found that 500 ml of solution produced 5000 pulmonary granulomas. The authors estimated that, in man subjected to the same i.v. fluid, 100 serial sections of lung would have to be examined to find a single granuloma [11]. I am not aware of careful autopsy studies seeking evidence of vascular bastosis from dialyzer or i.v. solution particulates in long-term dialysis patients.

SILICONE SPALLATION

The blood pump segment of older arterial blood tubing sets for hemodialysis was made of silicone rather than the now more commonly used PVC. The silicone spalls during the pumping process, causes vascular embolization, and is disseminated in the phagocytic system of hemodialysis patients. One patient developed pancytopenia due to splenic involvement, and required splenectomy [12]. In a study of 38 hemodialysis patients undergoing liver biopsy (and 31 other patients autopsied) within the hemodialysis patient group, silicone was found in 18 of the biopsied livers (47.4%), and in 22 (58%) of the livers at autopsy. The silicone caused varying degrees of granulomatous hepatitis in these patients. Of all 22 autopsied patients with silicone in the liver, silicone also was present in the spleens. It was found in the bone marrow of nine of these patients and in the lung of eight [13].

PLASTICIZERS

Both dialyzers and blood tubing sets are made of plastic. Diethylhexyl phthalate is a plasticizer commonly added to PVC blood tubing sets to achieve improved flexibility of the tubing at low temperatures. This plasticizer has been found to leach from the tubing to the patient's blood during hemodialysis [14], and has been implicated as the cause of necrotizing cutaneous vasculitis, and of a nonfatal hepatitis in hemodialysis patients [15].

STERILIZING AGENTS

A reaction product of the gas sterilant ethylene oxide, 2-chloroethanol, was found in a dialyzer and blood tubing set, and in the blood of a hemodialysis patient after a severe patient reaction shortly after initiating dialysis [16]. Formaldehyde, used by one manufacturer to sterilize hollow-fiber dialyzers until 1974 and incompletely purged from the dialyzer by then-recommended techniques, was the apparent cause of local burning sensations at the blood access site [17].

LIMULUS LYSATE-REACTIVE MATERIAL

New dialyzers, particularly those made with CUPROPHAN® membranes, may contain significant amounts of endotoxin, as determined by the limulus amebocyte lysate test [18, 19], and as confirmed by transmission electron-microscopic studies [20]. These contained endotoxins are extremely difficult to reduce to undetectable levels (less than 0.01 ng/ml). In one study, three successive days of blood compartment recirculation at 200 ml/min for 105 min was required to reduce the level of endotoxin by a factor of 10 in both hollow-fiber and parallel-plate dialyzers. Residual levels were still detectable (table 6-1). In another study, up to 13 dialyzer reprocessing cycles with a commercial reprocessing machine, each separated by 24 h of storage in 2.5% formaldehyde, were required to reduce endotoxin to undetectable levels [20]. In the same study, in some patients, never-used dialyzers purged of detectable levels of endotoxin did not provoke the significant neutropenia commonly observed early in dialysis in some patients. This observation suggests

Table 6-1. Leaching rate of endotoxin from the blood compartment of two new "pyrogen-free" dialyzers on successive days.

Day Hollow-fiber dialyzer	Leaching rate of endotoxin (ng/mim)	
	Parallel-plate dialyzer	
1	1.3	0.45
2	0.65	0.18
3	0.15	0.039

ᵃFrom Peterson et al. [19].

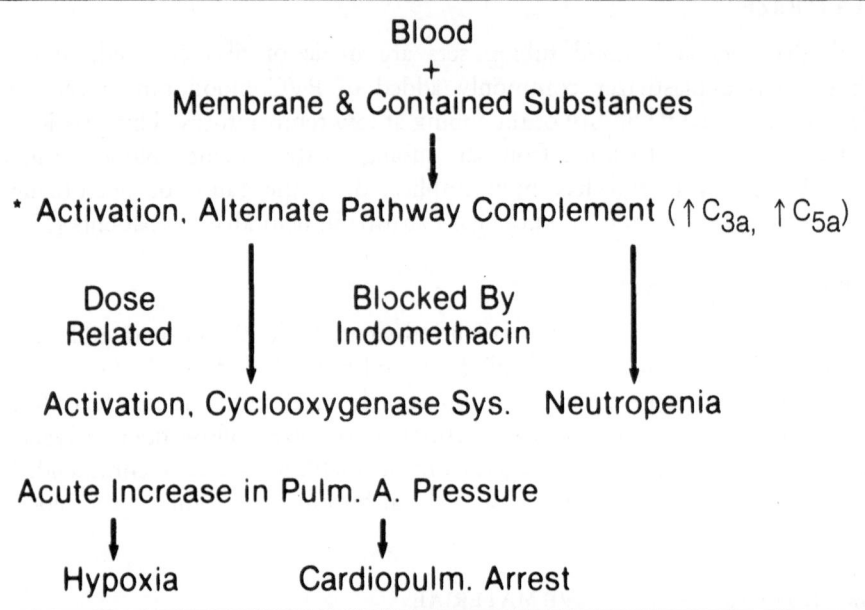

Figure 6-3. Schematic of early dialysis effects and dialyzer biocompatibility; a unifying concept of reactions between blood and dialysis membranes and/or contained substances. *Reduced in reprocessed dialyzers.

that in some patients it is the contained endotoxin, not the membrane itself, that causes the neutropenia.

MEMBRANE BIOCOMPATIBILITY

A rapidly growing literature indicates that blood from experimental animals, and from man, reacts with the dialysis membrane in a dose-related way to activate the alternate pathway of complement. CUPROPHAN® seems to provoke the most intense reaction, and polyacrylonitrile the least, with the cellulosic membranes in between. Used, reprocessed dialyzers cause less complement activation and neutropenia [20]. The activated complement leads both to the neutropenia first demonstrated in 1960 in dogs exposed to membrane artificial organs [21], and to activation of the cyclooxygenase system, first suggested by Walker and colleagues in 1983 [22]. The associated hemodynamic alterations, pulmonary hypertension, and decrease in cardiac output found in sheep exposed to dialysis membranes [22] may also occur in man and may, when particularly severe, play a role in the new dialyzer syndrome. A schematic illustrating these concepts is presented in figure 6-3. A more detailed discussion of complement activation with new and used dialyzer membranes may be found in chapter 10.

SAFETY OF USED DIALYZERS: GUIDELINES AND STANDARDS

In 1977, the Food and Drug Administration first published guidelines concerning the Reuse of Medical Disposable Devices (Compliance Policy Guide 7124.23), republished essentially unchanged as FDA Compliance Policy Guide 7124.16 in 1981. This Guide indicates that:

1. the institution or practitioner bears full responsibility for the safety and effectiveness of the reused device, and that
2. the institution or practitioner should be able to demonstrate that
   a. the device can be adequately cleaned and sterilized,
   b. the physical characteristics of the device will not be adversely affected, and
   c. the device remains safe and effective for its intended use.

These simple guidelines remain the keystone of successful dialyzer reuse in any facility and of the national practice of reuse that has become the standard in the United States.

The National Kidney Foundation published Interim Standards for Reuse of Hemodialyzers in 1982 [23], and Revised Standards for Reuse of Hemodialyzers in 1983 [24]. These are essentially outcome, not process, standards of safety, efficacy, esthetics, and informed patient consent. The Hemodialyzer Reuse Subcommittee of the Renal Disease and Detoxification Committee of the Association for the Advancement of Medical Instrumentation (AAMI) has been evolving a considerably more detailed, more process controlled "Recommended Practice for Reuse of Hemodialyzers" for the past two years. Their proposed recommendations are now available to the dialysis community; refer to chapter 12 for more information.

REPROCESSING OF USED DIALYZERS

Reprocessing of used dialyzers, in contrast to the manufacture of new dialyzers, is performed in perhaps 600 different facilities. Reprocessing techniques vary in at least some details in each facility. Although guidelines and standards exist as outlined above, no specific inspection of reuse practices, techniques, or outcomes by knowledgeable authorities exists. Compliance with techniques, quality control, and measures of quality assurance depends on the interest of the facility in providing excellent care for its patients, its economic interest in continuing the practice of reuse, and on its concern for legal liability for possible adverse patient effects related to reuse [25].

As with dialyzer manufacturing, successful dialyzer reprocessing requires strict quality control and quality assurance, including reprocessing specifications, process control, and sample validation studies. Unlike original manufacture, the reprocessed dialyzer must also be subjected to individual dialyzer efficacy (function), safety (disinfection and disinfectant removal), and esthetic tests before reuse. Specific techniques, function evaluation, disinfection, and quality control are discussed in considerable detail in chapters 2–5, respectively.

PATIENT HAZARDS OF REUSED DIALYZERS

The most commonly expressed concern of patients regarding reuse relates to the acute or long-term effects of formaldehyde, the agent most commonly used to disinfect reprocessed dialyzers. Reported acute toxicity includes discomfort at the site of the venous blood return [27], and the formation of anti-N-like antibodies resulting from early reuse practices involving dialyzer formaldehyde residuals of greater than 10 and up to 100 or more ppm, as discussed in detail in chapter 9. Hemolytic anemia has been reported as a consequence of formaldehyde release from new water filters installed in one dialysis unit [26]. Massive i.v. infusions of formaldehyde have occurred from failure to successfully purge dialysis machines or water distribution systems of formaldehyde used to disinfect this equipment before initiating dialysis. In one such episode, one patient died and several others were hospitalized with serious illnesses. I am not aware of any reports of massive infusions of formaldehyde related to dialyzer reuse.

Chronic toxicity from small, repeated i.v. infusions of formaldehyde has not been reported in man or animals. Dogs given 200 mg of formaldehyde per kilogram of body weight i.v. daily for 21 days evidenced no gross ill effects [28]. Inhalation exposure of 15 ppm, 6 h daily, five days a week for 16 months has been shown to produce nasopharyngeal carcinoma in rats [29]. This report continues to generate concern in the dialysis community, and has lent considerable impetus to the development and use of other agents for disinfecting reprocessed dialyzers, as mentioned in chapter 4.

It should be pointed out that pyrogenic reactions, sometimes severe or even fatal, used to be a significant problem in dialysis facilities. These reactions were usually due to excessive growth of gram-negative bacteria in water treatment equipment, the water distribution system, or the dialysis machines themselves [30]. Improved design of such equipment and frequent formaldehyde disinfection of the equipment have nearly eliminated this problem.

The practice of dialyzer reuse has not been associated with an increased incidence of hepatitis B in patients or staff [31], or with any increase in uremic peripheral neuropathy [32].

BACTEREMIA

Virtually all reported patient morbidity and mortality attributed to dialyzer reuse have resulted from inadequate disinfection and consequent gross bacterial contamination of the reprocessed dialyzer. During dialysis, large numbers of organisms, invariably water-borne bacteria, are then infused into the patient, usually resulting in clinical illness or death. In one episode, blood samples of 16 of 33 patients grew *Pseudomonas cepacia* following inadvertent omission of a "step of the sterilization and storage procedure," a quality control omission. Of the 16 patients, 13 became clinically ill. In one patient, the bacteria caused infection in a polycystic kidney, resulting in a three-month illness [33]. In another report from a center reusing coils and using benzalkonium chloride as a "sterilizing agent," *Pseudomonas aeruginosa* was cultured from the blood of ten (59%) of 17 patients during 18 of 201 dialyses, and one patient died of *Pseudomonas* endocarditis [34].

Nontuberculous mycobacteria, present by culture in a high percent of samples of municipal water supplies, may multiply in dialysis water treatment and distribution equipment, and are highly resistant to the effects of most disinfectants, including formaldehyde [35]. These characteristics of mycobacteria, combined with inadequate quality control of levels of formaldehyde used as the disinfectant for reprocessing dialyzers, resulted in 27 cases of nontuberculous mycobacterial infection among 140 patients at two outpatient hemodialysis centers in Baton Rouge, Louisiana [36, 37]. Serious clinical illnesses were associated with these infections. Although the extent to which these infections contributed to patient mortality was not immediately apparent, 13 of the 27 patients died within a year of their infection. Additional discussion of water bacteria and their potential role in dialysis morbidity can be found in chapter 4.

MORTALITY: NEW VERSUS USED DIALYZERS

It is obvious from the foregoing discussion that patient deaths have been directly attributable to problems with both new and used dialyzers. Those obviously attributable to new dialyzers are largely from the new dialyzer syndrome; those obviously attributable to used dialyzers resulted from inadequate disinfection, bacteremia, and subsequent clinical infection.

It is also apparent from the foregoing discussion that more subtle and more long-term morbidity and/or mortality relating primarily to chronic patient exposure to the residua of manufacturing or of reprocessing, may result from new or used dialyzers. There are no prospective studies to provide data regarding such morbidity. Indeed, in view of the many morbid and mortal events that occur in dialysis patients, unless such exposure were a substantial factor in patient morbidity, it is highly unlikely that a prospective study would reveal a significant difference in patient mortality attributable solely to reuse or non-reuse of dialyzers. Retrospective, epidemiologic data from European dialysis centers (see chapter 1, table 1-1) fail to provide convincing data for an effect of dialyzer reuse on patient mortality [37]. (See also chapter 7.)

CONCLUSIONS

1. Driven initially by economic considerations, and more recently by both economic factors and medical considerations of biocompatibility, dialyzer reuse has become the standard of practice in the United States.
2. Patient morbidity and mortality, acute and perhaps chronic, may be associated with the use of both new and reprocessed dialyzers.
3. In view of the fact that over 10,000,000 hemodialyses are now performed annually in this country, reported significant morbidity or mortality related to either new or reused dialyzers is extremely small.
4. It is incumbent on the entire community of dialysis interests to freely acknowledge potential and actual problems with both new and reprocessed dialyzers, and to continue to work to minimize or eliminate these problems.

REFERENCES

1. Kennedy AC, Linton AI, Renfrew S, Luke RG, Dinwoodie A: The pathogenesis and prevention of cerebral dysfunction during dialysis. Lancet 1:790−793, 1964.
2. Rosen SM, O'Connor K, Shaldon S: Haemodialysis disequilibrium. Br Med J 5410:672−675, 1964.
3. Kjellstrand CM, Alfrey AC, Eaton JW, Friedman EA, Ginn HE, Hull AR, Odgen DA: Toxicity of materials and medications used in dialysis. Trans Am Soc Artif Inter Organs 24:764−769, 1978.
4. Ogden DA: New-dialyzer syndrome. N Engl J Med 302:1262−1263, 1980.
5. Bok DV, Pascual L, Herberger C, Sawyer R, Levine NW: Effect of multiple use dialyzers on intradialytic symptoms. Proc Dial Transplant Forum 10:92−99, 1980.
6. Kant KS, Pollak VE, Cathey M, Goetz D, Berlin R: Multiple use of dialyzers: safety and efficacy. Kidney Int 19:728−738, 1981.
7. Popli S, Ing TS, Daugirdas JT, Kheirbek AO, Viol GW, Vilbar RM, Gandhi VC: Severe reactions to CUPROPHAN capillary dialyzers. Artif Organs 6:312−315, 1982.
8. Ing TS, Daugirdas JT, Popli S, Gandhi VC: First-use syndrome with cuprammonium cellulose dialyzers. Int J Artif Organs 6:235−239, 1983.
9. Villarroel F, Ciarkowski AA: A survey of hypersensitivity reactions in hemodialysis. Artif Organs 9:231−238, 1985.
10. Sarrut S, Nezelof C: Une complication de la therapeutique intraveineuse. Presse Med 68:375−377, 1960.
11. Garvan JM, Gunner BW: The harmful effects of particles in intravenous fluids. Med J Aust 2:1−6, 1964.
12. Bommer J, Ritz E, Waldherr R: Silicone-induced splenomegaly. N Engl J Med 305:1077−1079, 1981.
13. Leong AS, Disney APS, Gove DW: Spallation and migration of silicone from blood-pump tubing in patients on hemodialysis. N Engl J Med 306:135−140, 1982.
14. Ono K, Tatsukawa R, Wakimoto T: Migration of plasticizer from hemodialysis blood tubing. JAMA 234:948−949, 1975.
15. Neergaard J, Nielsen B, Faurby V, Christensen DH, Neilsen OF: Plasticizers in P.V.C. and the occurrence of hepatitis in a haemodialysis unit. Scand J Urol Nephrol 5:141−145, 1971.
16. Gutch CF, Eskelson CD, Ziegler E, Ogden DA: 2-Chloroethanol as a toxic residue in dialysis supplies sterilized with ethylene oxide. Dial Transplant 5:21−25, 1976.
17. Ogden DA, Myers LE, Eskelson CD, Ziegler EJ: Iatrogenic administration of formaldehyde to hemodialysis patients. Proc Dial Transplant Forum 3:141−146, 1973.
18. Deane N: Dialyzer reuse and therapeutic effect. AAMI Technology Assessment Report: reuse of disposables 6-83, 1983, pp 24−28.
19. Petersen NJ, Carson JA, Favero MS: Bacterial endotoxin in new and reused hemodialyzers: a potential cause of endotoxemia. Trans Am Soc Artif Intern Organs 27:155−160, 1981.

20. Pizzaconi VB, Dorson WJ, Breillat J, Hyde GM, Aniuk LM, Walsh SA, Bland LA, Brady RL: Factors affecting complement activation and neutropenia during dialysis using cuprophane membranes. Am Soc Artif Intern Organs J 7:64−73, 1984.
21. Mito M, Nishimura A, Sumiyoshi S, Kawai M, Nose Y, Yoshimoto C: On extracorporeal circulation of membrane artificial organs (liver and kidney). Sogoigaku 17:538, 1960.
22. Walker JF, Lindsay RM, Peters SD, Sibbald WJ, Linton AL: A sheep model to examine the cardiopulmonary manifestations of blood dialyzer interactions. Am Soc Artif Intern Organs J 6:123−130, 1983.
23. National Kidney Foundation: Interim standards for reuse of hemodialyzers. Am J Kidney Dis 2:315, 1982.
24. National Kidney Foundation: Revised standards for reuse of hemodialyzers. Am J Kidney Dis 3:466−468, 1984.
25. Hallquist SG: Legal consequences of disposable dialyzer reuse. Am J Law Med 8:1−25, 1982.
26. Orringer EP, Mattern WD: Formaldehyde-induced hemolysis during chronic hemodialysis. N Engl J Med 294:1416−1420, 1976.
27. Orloff MJ, Peskin GW: The effect of formaldehyde on experimental ammonia intoxication. Surg Forum 10:295−300, 1960.
28. Formaldehyde: evidence of carcinogenicity. NIOSH Current Intelligence Bulletin 34, DHEW (NIOSH) Publication no. 81-111, 15 April 1981.
29. Petersen NJ, Boyer KM, Carson LA, Favero MS: Pyrogenic reactions from inadequate disinfection of a dialysis fluid distribution system. Dial Transplant 7:52−60, 1978.
30. Favero MS, Deane N, Leger RT, Sosin AE: Effect of multiple use of dialyzers on hepatitis B incidence in patients and staff. JAMA 245:166−167, 1981.
31. Sosin AE, Iyer K, Bemis JA, Rigney JH, Deane N: Uremic neuropathy and multiple usage of dialyzers. Artif Organs [Suppl] 2:456, 1978.
32. Kuehnel E, Lundh H: Outbreak of *Pseudomonas cepacia* bacteremia related to contaminated reused coils. Dial Transplant 5:44−48, 66, 1976.
33. Wagnild JP, McDonald P, Craig WA, Johnson C, Hanley M, Uman SJ, Ramgopal V, Beisne GJ: *Pseudomonas aeruginosa* bacteremia in a dialysis unit. II. Relationship to reuse of coils. Am J Med 62:672−676, 1977.
34. Carson LA, Petersen NJ, Favero MS, Aguero SM: Growth characteristics of atypical mycobacteria in water and their comparative resistance to disinfectants. Appl Environ Microbiol 36:839−46, 1978.
35. Morbidity and mortality weekly report, US Department of Health and Human Services/ Public Health Service 32:244, 13 May 1983.
36. Bingaman C: Water treatment procedures and formaldehyde-resistant mycobacteria challenge two Baton Rouge dialysis facilities. Contemp Dial 4(6):34−49, 1983.
37. Wing AJ, Brunner FP, Brynger HOA, Chantler C, Donckerwolcke RA, Gurland JH, Jacobs C, Selwood NH: Mortality and morbidity of reusing dialyzers. Br Med J 2:853−855, 1978.

7. USE AND REUSE OF DIALYZERS IN EUROPE

SABRI CHALLAH
ANTONY J. WING
FELIX P. BRUNNER
HANS O.A. BRYNGER
R. OULES
NEVILLE H. SELWOOD

The European Dialysis and Transplant Association—European Renal Association (EDTA—ERA) Registry collects data on patients receiving treatment for end-stage renal disease (ESRD) throughout Europe. Annual returns from 32 countries are made to the Registry by means of both a center and individual patient questionnaire. For the past 13 years, detailed information on use and reuse of dialyzers has been included in the patient questionnaire. Clinicians are asked to record the code number for the type of dialyzer most frequently used during the previous 12 months, and state the number of reuses, if any, achieved on average by each individual patient. The Registry currently maintains codes for over 300 different types of dialyzers, as well as separate codes for hemofilters.

Data on hemodialysis practice including reuse of dialyzers have been published in the past [1]. In 1977, the Registry undertook a special study to look at the impact of reuse on mortality and morbidity among ESRD patients in the United Kingdom [2].

USE OF DIALYZERS IN EUROPE

The pattern of use of dialyzers in Europe has changed dramatically over the last decade. Figure 7-1 shows the percentage of patients using each of the four main groups of dialyzer—nondisposable (Kiil), parallel flow, coil and capillary (hollow fiber)—between 1975 and 1983 in all countries reporting to the Registry. There has been a steady decline in the proportion of patients using

Deane, Wineman, and Bemis (eds.): GUIDE TO REPROCESSING OF HEMODIALYSERS.
© 1986. Martinus Nijhoff Publishing. All rights reserved.

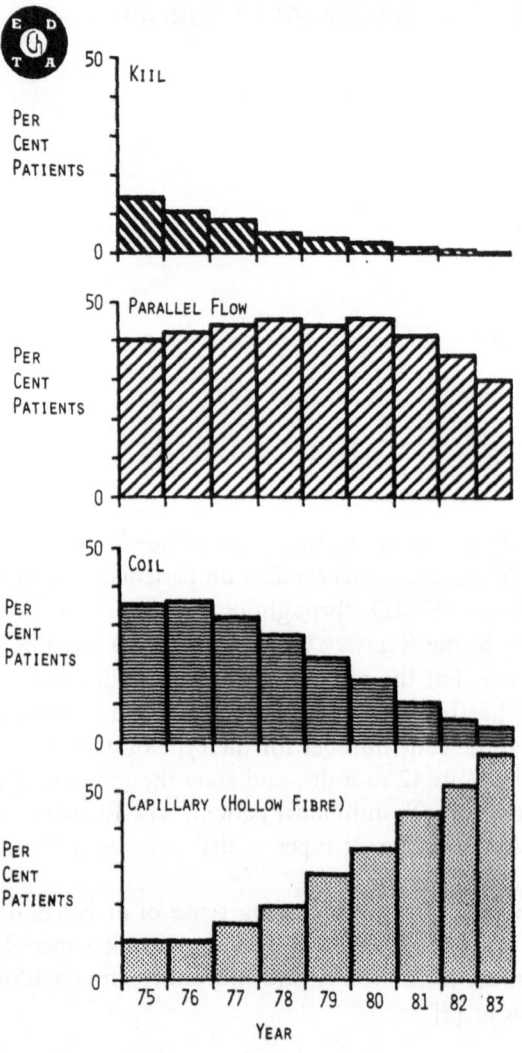

Figure 7-1. The percentage of patients using each of the four main groups of dialyzers in the years 1975–1983 throughout Europe.

the nondisposable (Kiil) and coil dialyzers, of which the majority were in France and the United Kingdom. In the same year, coil dialyzers were used by just over 5% of subjects. In contrast, capillary dialyzers accounted for 62% of use, having risen progressively from just over 10% in 1975. Almost half the patients in Europe used parallel-flow dialyzers between 1978 and 1980, but this figure had declined to just under a third by 1983.

The type of dialyzer used differs greatly between countries. Kiil dialyzers are no longer used in 12 out of the 19 countries shown in table 7-1. In

Table 7-1. The percentage of patients using each of the four main groups of dialyzer in 1983 by country.

Country	Non disposable parallel flow (%)	Disposable (%)		
		Parallel flow	Coil	Hollow fiber
Austria	0	17.3	0.9	81.8
Belgium	0	41.3	0.6	58.1
Czechoslovakia	0	4.7	89.6	5.6
German Dem Republic	0	0.4	0	99.6
Denmark	0	52.4	0	47.6
Fed Rep Germany	0.1	19.8	0.1	80.0
Finland	0	54.4	0	45.6
France	2.2	27.6	0.2	70.0
Greece	0	28.1	8.7	63.2
Hungary	0	42.5	27.1	30.4
Italy	0.1	62.1	0.8	37.0
Netherlands	0	46.5	0	53.5
Norway	0	15.4	0	84.6
Poland	0.3	24.6	69.5	5.6
Spain	0.2	18.0	11.7	70.1
Sweden	0	35.0	0	65.0
Switzerland	0	34.1	4.9	61.0
United Kingdom	6.4	42.7	2.5	48.4
Yugoslavia	0.1	43.5	8.4	48.1

Czechoslovakia and Poland, coil dialyzers were used by the majority of patients in 1983, while in Finland, Italy, and Hungary the majority used the disposable parallel-flow type. In the remaining 15 nations the use of capillary dialyzers predominated. There are no obvious explanations for these differences between European countries.

REUSE OF DIALYZERS IN EUROPE

In 1982, just over 10% of patients reported to the EDTA−ERA Registry practiced reuse of dialyzers; this had fallen to 9.2% in the following year, about half the 1976 level [2]. The practice of reuse had been comparable to the United States in 1978, when it was estimated that 15.7% of patients were reusing dialyzers [3].

Trends in reuse for the different groups of dialyzers between 1975 and 1983 are shown in figure 7-2. Among the few patients still using nondisposable (Kiil) dialyzers, about 50% still reused in 1983, compared with 70% two years previously. Reuse of disposable capillary and parallel-flow dialyzers leveled off at around 10% in 1982 and 1983, while the figure for the coil type rose slightly in 1983 to 15% of patients.

Figure 7-3 shows the percentage of patients using dialyzers between 1975 and 1979, according to whether they were treated at home or in hospital. Reuse was much more common among patients on home treatment, but the pattern seems to be changing slowly.

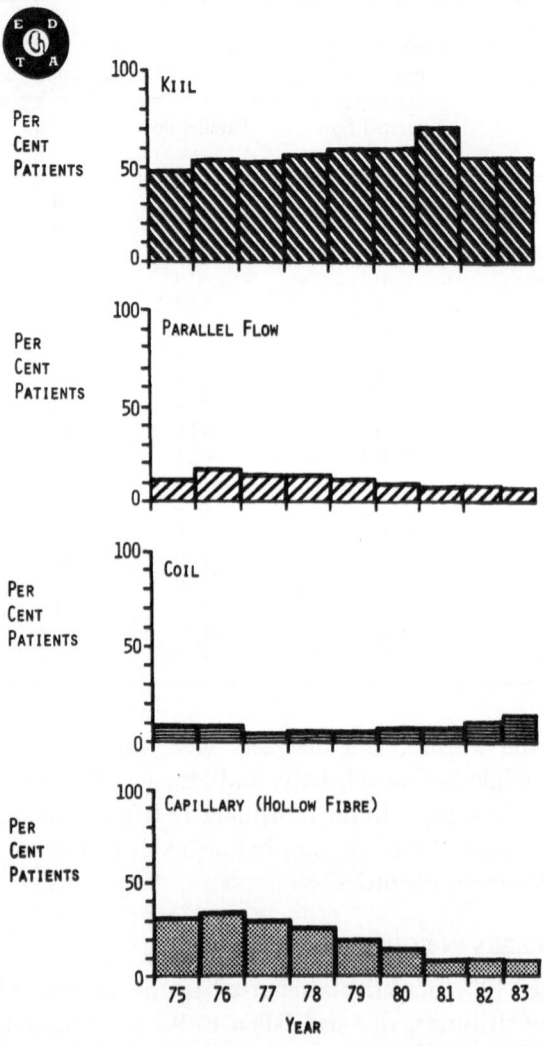

Figure 7-2. The percentage of patients reusing each of the four main groups of dialyzers between 1975 and 1983 throughout Europe.

Although reuse practice still varies greatly among different European countries, the range appears to be narrowing. In 1980, for example, the proportion of patients reusing ranged from zero in Finland and Greece to 99% in Poland. In 1983 every nation reported some reuse, although as low as 0.1% in some cases. Poland still led with 75.9% of patients reusing (table 7-2).

It is difficult to see a common thread in the trends described for individual countries. In those which are traditionally heavy reusers such as Poland and the United Kingdom, it is clear that a movement against reuse has emerged. In the four years 1980–1983, the percentage of patients reusing in the United

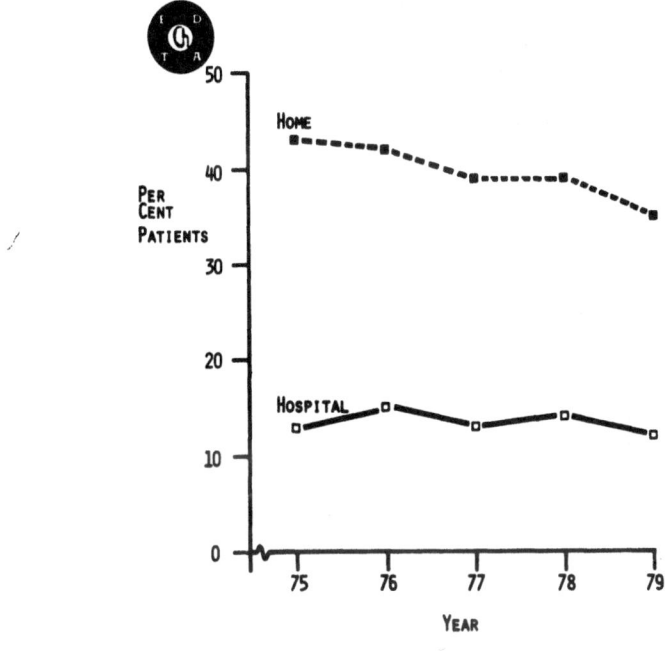

Figure 7-3. Comparison of reuse of dialyzers in home and hospital patients between 1975 and 1979.

Table 7-2. The percentage of patients reusing dialyzers in 1980–1983 by countries: countries are ranked according to reuse practice in 1983.

Country	1980 (%)	1981 (%)	1982 (%)	1983 (%)
Poland	99.0	84.0	77.5	75.9
United Kingdom	61.9	62.8	57.0	35.4
Switzerland	34.4	29.3	37.1	34.8
Hungary	15.4	17.5	26.4	22.3
Belgium	7.7	8.5	9.2	10.2
France	16.9	11.9	11.4	9.7
Norway	10.3	6.5	4.2	9.0
Denmark	3.8	6.0	5.2	6.9
Austria	0.2	0.3	0.2	5.4
Czechoslovakia	2.7	1.1	12.6	5.4
Yugoslavia	2.2	0.8	1.6	4.3
Spain	6.7	5.1	4.8	3.5
Fed Rep Germany	1.7	2.1	2.2	2.4
Finland	0	0.9	0	1.5
Italy	1.5	0.6	0.6	1.3
Sweden	0.1	0.7	0.7	1.2
Greece	0	0	0	0.4
German Dem Rep	74.5	1.4	2.3	0.2
Netherlands	1.0	0.2	1.0	0.1

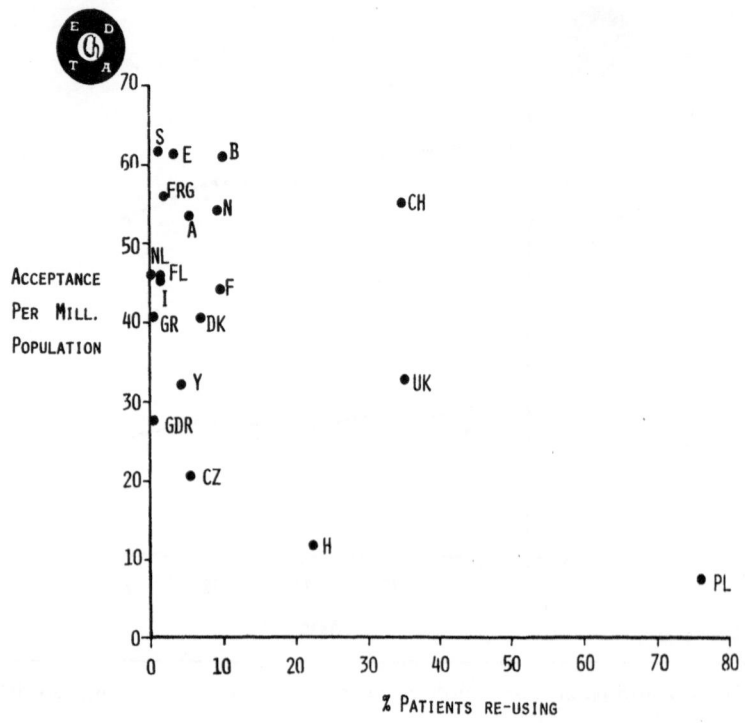

Figure 7-4. The relationship between acceptance rates onto dialysis and transplant programs per million population and the percentage of patients reusing dialyzers in 19 European countries:
S, Sweden; E, Spain; B, Belgium; FRG, The Federal Republic of Germany; CH, Switzerland; A, Austria; N, Norway; NL, The Netherlands; FL, Finland; F, France; I, Italy; GR, Greece; DK, Denmark; Y, Yugoslavia; UK, The United Kingdom; GDR, The German Democratic Republic; CZ, Czechoslovakia; H, Hungary; and PL, Poland.

Kingdom fell from 61.9 to 34.5. Even more striking are figures from the German Democratic Republic that showed a decline from 74.5% to 0.2% over the same period, with capillary dialyzers used in over 95% of patients. This change is probably associated with the shift to domestic manufacture of dialyzers. Among some low reusers such as the Federal Republic of Germany and Sweden there was a slight increase while in others such as Spain and France there was a decrease in the practice of reuse.

It is equally difficult to explain the pattern of reuse observed across Europe. No single factor can account for different policies in individual countries. Undoubtedly, in the United Kingdom and Poland, a large part of the drive toward reuse is due to economic factors. These countries have low acceptance rates for renal replacement therapy and savings that may accrue from reuse make it possible to treat more patients. However, this explanation alone does not suffice. Figure 7-4 shows the relationship between acceptance

Table 7-3. The average number of reuses by main group of dialyzer and country in 1983.

Country	Non disposable parallel flow	Disposable		
		Parallel flow	Coil	Hollow fiber
Austria	—	2	—	2
Belgium	—	4	5	4
.Czechoslovakia	—	1	1	1
German Dem Rep	—	—	—	1
Denmark	—	2	—	—
Fed Rep Germany	3	2	—	4
Finland	—	1	—	1
France	4	2	3	2
Greece	—	2	—	2
Hungary	—	—	—	3
Italy	—	2	—	2
Netherlands	—	—	—	2
Norway	—	1	—	1
Poland	—	3	4	2
Spain	—	1	3	8
Sweden	—	1	—	1
Switzerland	—	2	2	2
United Kingdom	3	3	—	3
Yugoslavia	—	1	1	1

rates for dialysis and transplantation and reuse practice, expressed as a percentage of patients reusing, in 19 European countries. There is no correlation between the two, and it seems that reuse policy must be influenced by a variety of factors, which vary in importance from nation to nation.

Table 7-3 shows the average number of reuses by type of dialyzer and country in 1983. In many cases the numbers of patients involved are small. The mean number of reuses of the disposable parallel-flow type range from one in a number of countries to four in Belgium; an average of eight reuses in 229 patients was reported from Spain for hollow-fiber dialyzers.

MORBIDITY AND MORTALITY RELATED TO REUSE

Information on morbidity associated with reuse of dialyzers has been published by the EDTA Registry [2] and elsewhere [3]. In 1976, the Registry carried out a special survey in the United Kingdom renal units to look specifically into this question. Of the 33 centers in which disposable dialyzers had been reused, 13 reported pyrexial reactions and three cases of bacteremia due to reuse. The results of the study, which relate to morbidity, are shown in table 7-4, together with those from a similar survey of 642 units in the United States, of which 107 reported reuse [3].

Although both the American and the EDTA surveys indicated the number of units that had reported complications associated with reuse, no results were presented on the incidence of these problems in non-reusing centers. In the absence of such a comparison, it is difficult to draw conclusions about

Table 7-4. Adverse reactions reported from reuse of dialyzers in studies from the United Kingdom and the United States.

United Kingdom	United States
Pyrexial reaction, bacteremia	Pyrexial reaction, bacteremia
Incidents with sterilizing agents	Formalin reactions
Mechanical problems, e.g., membrane rupture, loss of dialyzer clearance	Technical problems with storage or loss of dialyzer clearance
Development of anti-N antibodies	Development of anti-N antibodies
	Possible spread of hepatitis
	Dialyzer used on wrong patient

morbidity specifically associated with reuse. No deaths were attributed to reuse in either survey.

There is no evidence that reuse adversely affects patient survival [1]. A study by the Registry compared the one-year survival of reusers and non-reusers commencing renal replacement therapy in the year of the report [1]. There was no significant difference in the one-year survival of the two groups: 93.2% of reusers vs 91.2% of non-reusers. Caution should be exercised in generalizing from these results, since confounding variables, other than age, were not considered. The question has also been examined by comparing survival in countries with low versus high reuse practice [2]; no unfavorable effect on survival could be detected from reuse. The character of patients on treatment differs greatly between countries, however, even within cohorts of similar age. It is particularly problematic to compare countries having high reuse and low acceptance rates such as the United Kingdom and those having low reuse and high acceptance rates such as the Federal Republic of Germany. The Registry has reported that patients with multisystem disease are underrepresented in the dialysis and transplant populations of those countries having a low acceptance rate for renal replacement therapy.

More sophisticated studies of the effects of reuse on morbidity and mortality are required. At the present time we can say that the available information has failed to demonstrate any severe harmful effects of dialyzer reuse on patient survival.

REFERENCES

1. Jacobs C, Brunner FP, Chantler C, Donckerwolcke RA, Gurland HJ, Hathway RA, Selwood NH, Wing AJ: Combined reports on regular dialysis and transplantation in Europe. VII. Proc Eur Dial Transplant Assoc 14:3–69, 1977.
2. Wing AJ, Brunner FP, Brynger H, Chantler C, Donckerwolcke RA, Gurland HJ, Jacobs C, Selwood NH: Mortality and morbidity of re-using dialysers. Br Med J 2:853–855, 1978.
3. Deane N, Blagg CR, Bower J, De Palma J, Gutch C, Kanter A, Ogden D, Sadler J, Siemsen N, Teehan B, Sosin A: A survey of dialyzer reuse practice in the United States. Dial Transplant 7:1128–1130, 1978.

8. TECHNICAL ASPECTS OF REUSE IN EUROPE

NICHOLAS A. HOENICH
T.H.J. GOODSHIP
MICHAEL K. WARD
S. RINGOIR

The feasibility of maintenance hemodialysis as a mode of treatment for chronic renal failure was established in the early 1960s [1]. By the end of that decade, 217 centers in Europe were treating 2816 patients by this technique. Patients used principally the Kiil type nondisposable (56.4%) and coil (26.2%) disposable dialyzers. Although both were reused, the rationale behind their reuse differed. In the case of the Kiil and its later multipoint variants [2], reuse was on the basis of convenience rather than cost since such dialyzers were built for use on each occasion. After building, they required sterilization, which was undertaken by the filling of the blood and dialysate compartments with formaldehyde and, prior to each use, the formaldehyde was rinsed out. As these procedures were time consuming, reuse of such devices became common and grew from the desire to reduce the time spent in assembling and preparing the devices. In the case of the disposable coil dialyzer, which was supplied in a presterilized package, cost was the primary consideration in reusing [3].

During the next two decades, acceptance rates of new patients increased, the strategies of treatments altered and, by 1982, 1456 centers in Europe were treating 53,874 patients. Since the basis for reuse of hemodialyzers had already been established, the practice continued.

THE DEMOGRAPHY OF REUSE IN EUROPE

The pattern of hemodialyzer use in Europe over the period 1975–1983 is shown in table 8-1. During this period, the use of nondisposable flat-plate hemodialyzers declined so that in 1983 less than 1% of the patients treated were using this type of dialyzer. Over the same period, while the use of coil dialyzers declined, there was a marked growth in the use of hollow-fiber and disposable flat-plate devices.

The European Dialysis and Transplant Association–European Renal Association (EDTA–ERA) analyzed the pattern of dialyzer reuse in Europe during the period 1975–1982 according to dialyzer type, dialysis site (center or home), and country [4] (see chapter 7). During this period, reuse was confined principally to nondisposable flat-plate dialyzers with more than 50% of the patients on this type of dialyzer reusing them in 1981, compared with 10% or less for other types in the same year. The reuse of capillary dialyzers declined as their popularity increased. The practice of reusing parallel-flow and coil dialyzers changed little between 1975 and 1981.

These figures represent the average and encompass returns from 32 countries participating in the EDTA–ERA registry. A wide variation in the popularity of the practice of reuse exists.

In 1981, reuse was most prevalent in Bulgaria, where 97% of patients treated (384) reused. In Poland it was practiced by 84% of the patients treated (426), while 63% of the United Kingdom dialysis population (2819) reused. In Poland and Bulgaria, the practice was confined principally to nondisposable dialyzers while, in the United Kingdom, reuse of nondisposable flat-plate dialyzers was most dominant with 83% of the patients treated by such dialyzer reusing. The practice in other countries varied from virtually no reuse (0–1% of the patients treated in Italy, the Netherlands, the Federal

Table 8-1. Use of hemodialyzers in Europe showing percentage of patients reported as using the dialyzer most frequently that year.

	Hemodialyzer type					No. of patients treated
			Disposable			
Year	Non disposable flat plate	Flat plate	Coil	Hollow fiber	Hemofilter	
1975	13.7	40.2	35.2	10.4		25862
1976	11	42.2	35.8	10.4		30411
1977	8.7	43.2	31.4	14.6		34581
1978	6.4	46	27.7	19.8		38261
1979	4.7	44.7	22.3	28.3		39728
1980	3.1	45.7	16.6	34.6	1.2	53519
1981	2.1	41.1	11.1	43.8	1.7	61342
1982	1.2	37.1	6.9	52.6	2.0	69876
1983	0.8	31.2	5.3	60.6	2.1	75237

From the EDTA Registry.

Table 8-2. Use of hemodialyzers in the United Kingdom showing percentage of patients reported as using the dialyzer most frequently that year.

		Hemodialyzer type				No. of patients treated
			Disposable			
Year	Non disposable flat plate	Flat plate	Coil	Hollow fiber	Hemofilter	
1975	70	8.9	13.1	10.9		2615
1976	61.6	13.3	13.4	11.6		2891
1977	56	16.8	12.1	22.2		3170
1978	41.6	22.8	10.7	19.6		3594
1979	38.5	28.6	8.7	23.9		3876
1980	31.4	30.7	8.7	29		4215
1981	20.5	36.5	7.8	35		4491
1982	9.6	41.1	6.7	41.9	0.2	4611
1983	6.4	42.6	2.5	48.3	0.1	4271

From the EDTA Registry.

Republic of Germany, Sweden, Czechoslovakia, and Yugoslavia) to 29% (Switzerland).

It would appear from these figures that European countries with small treatment groups and those with adequate funding for the treatment program tend not to reuse. As the treatment population or the cost of treatment increases, it is possible that economic considerations play an increasingly important role in reuse and the practice then grows.

In the United Kingdom, the use of dialyzer types differed from the rest of Europe (table 8-2). In spite of their decline in use, nondisposable dialyzers continued to be used by 6.4% of the patients treated in 1983 (275 patients). Paralleling the European figures, coil usage also declined while the use of disposable parallel-flow and hollow-fiber dialyzers grew. The use of hollow-fiber dialyzers nevertheless remained below the European average.

Wing et al., in their review of hemodialyzer reuse in the United Kingdom in 1976 [5], showed that 65.6% of the patients treated with nondisposable dialyzers (1785 patients) and 49.6% of those using disposable dialyzers (1109 patients) reused. By 1981 the number of patients using nondisposable dialyzers had fallen to 921, but 83% of these patients continued to reuse. Patients using disposable dialyzers had risen to 3566 and, of these, 56% were reusing, irrespective of dialyzer type.

To assess the current situation, 61 dialysis centers in the United Kingdom were queried on their reuse practices. Of the 53 (87%) centers replying to the questionnaire, 17 were actively reusing, ten had stopped in the preceding year, and 26 had stopped prior to this. In the centers practicing reuse, a total of 1250 patients were treated compared with 2175 in the centers not reusing. Of the patients being treated by centers that were reusing, 498 (40%) and 748

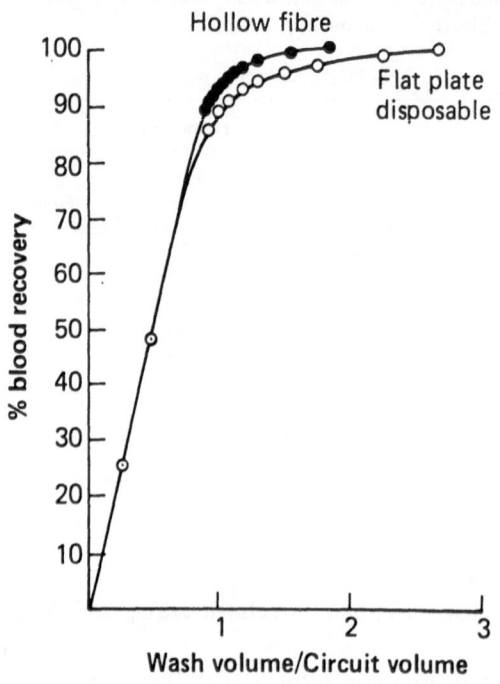

Figure 8-1. Blood recovery curves for flat-plate and hollow-fiber disposable hemodialyzers.

(60%) were treated in the hospital and home, respectively, with 48% of the hospital group reusing compared with 73% of the home patients.

THE REUSE PROCEDURE

The technique of reuse, the practice in which hemodialyzers are used for multiple dialyses of the same patient, may be subdivided into four distinct steps: first, the rinsing of the dialyzer at the termination of dialysis, followed by cleaning, and then sterilization to allow its storage between uses. The preparation of the dialyzer prior to subsequent use is the final stage of the procedure. (See chapter 2.)

At the termination of dialysis, the blood contained in the extracorporeal circuit is normally returned to the patient by rinsing of the extracorporeal circuit with saline. Other rinsing solutions such as isotonic dextrose may also be employed. The blood remaining in the circuit at the termination of treatment comprises two distinct components. The first is the fluid blood component, whose magnitude is related to the dialyzer design, the heparin administered, the volume of the rinsing solution used, and the technique of rinse back. Figure 8-1 shows that the majority of this blood may be rinsed out of the device, provided a sufficiently large volume of rinsing solution is used at the termination of dialysis. The second component is the clotted

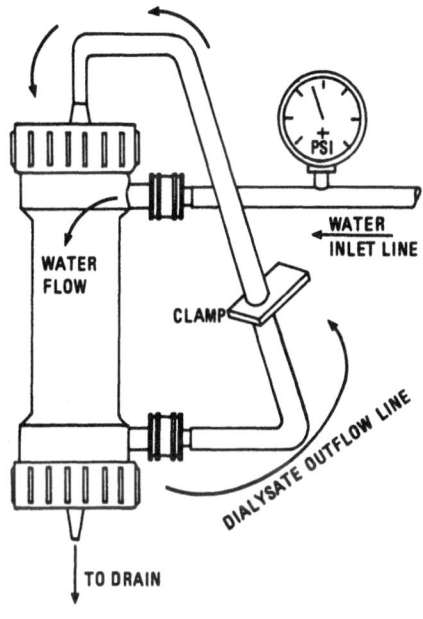

Figure 8-2. Hydraulic circuit for manual reuse of hollow-fiber hemodialyzers.

residue that has formed during treatment in spite of heparinization, the removal of which may only be achieved by the physical disruption of the clot.

The cleaning phase of the reuse procedure consists of two components: first, a period of prolonged flushing usually with tap water that may or may not be treated, followed by or coupled with chemical cleaning. Chemical cleaning may be performed by the use of sodium hypochlorite [6], hydrogen peroxide [6], or by a number of new agents such as RENALIN®, a stabilized mixture of hydrogen peroxide, peracetic acid mixed with acetic acid, CYDEX® (glutaraldehyde) and WAREXIN® (monoxychlorosene), a tetradecyl-benzene-sulfonate-hypochlorous acid complex, or SPORICIDIN-HD® a synergized glutaraldehyde phenate solution [7]. Some of these can also be used as sterilants, but formaldehyde remains the most widely used.

After the storage period between uses, the dialyzer is prepared for subsequent use by the flushing of the sterilant from the blood and dialysate compartments. Saline is most widely used for the rinsing of the blood compartment, while the dialysate compartment is rinsed either with tap water or dialysis fluid. The aim of this predialysis flushing is to remove the sterilant from the respective compartments and to render the dialyzer suitable for use. These components, which are summarized in table 8-3, may be used in any combination, giving rise to a wide range of techniques. Furthermore, many of the components of reuse have been automated or made semiautoma-

112

Table 8-3. Agents that may be used in the reprocessing of hemodialyzers.

Postdialysis rinsing	Postdialysis cleaning	Sterilization	Predialysis blood compartment	Rinsing dialysate compartment
Saline		Formaldehyde	Saline	Dialysis fluid
	Treated tap water	Glutaraldehyde		Treated tapwater
Treated tap water	Dialysis fluid	Sodium hypochlorite		
Dialysis fluid	Chemical			
Chemical		Other		

tic, enabling them to be adapted for multiple dialyzer reprocessing as well as for individual use. It is not possible, nor is it proposed, to review these techniques in detail since they are covered elsewhere in this monograph.

Our own experiences when reusing hemodialyzers have been confined to the three methods that are described in detail below.

Manual technique for single patient use

This technique is based on that described by Craske et al. [8] and is suitable for use with hollow-fiber hemodialyzers. The circuit shown in figure 8-2 is used; while our technique is for a single dialyzer, it may be adapted easily to multiple dialyzer reprocessing.

Following the termination of dialysis immediately after disconnection from the patient, the dialyzer is rinsed with room temperature reverse osmosis water at a pressure of 15 psi. During this rinsing process, which lasts 8–10 min, the dialysate outflow line is periodically clamped. The positive pressure thus generated forces water across the fiber wall, loosening blood products adhering to the fibers. When the pressure is released, water flows through the fibers, flushing out the blood components. This procedure is repeated until the dialyzer is completely clear of blood residue. It is then tested and filled with formalin (5% formalin = 2% formaldehyde) prior to storage.

Automated technique for single patient use

Single patient automated reuse systems are suitable for patients who dialyze at home. Fitzcharles et al. [9] described one such system based on the modification of the Dylade DS single patient proportionating system, while Jeffrey (personal communication) adapted the Cobe Centry 11 machine to enable it to reprocess dialyzers in the home. In these systems, which are equally suitable for both flat-plate and hollow-fiber dialyzers, the fluid produced by the proportionating system is used to rinse the dialyzer and, as both the proportionating systems are chemically sterilized, they are used to sterilize the dialyzer and the blood lines if so desired. Use of such systems clearly is confined to dialysis patients using these proportionating systems. For others, free-standing systems are more appropriate (several such systems have been described in the literature [10–12]). Our experience is confined to one such system described in 1977 and produced by ABG Semca (ABG Semca type 704S), which is suitable for single patient use with both hollow-fiber and flat-plate designs [12].

The system rinses the dialyzer's blood compartment with sodium hypochlorite (0.5%) automatically. This rinsing period lasts 12 min during which the flow through the blood compartment (500 ml/min) is pulsed. This chemical rinse of the blood compartment is followed by a formalin rinse lasting 6 min, after which the blood and dialysate compartments of the dialyzer are filled with 2% formaldehyde. The dialyzer may then be removed from the system or, if used at home, it may be kept connected to the system, which has the facility to reuse blood lines as well as the dialyzer. Prior to subsequent use, automatic rinsing of the dialyzer's dialysate compartment with a water flow of 1 liter/min for a period of 10 min may be performed.

Automated technique for multiple patient use

The Texas Medical Devices ADR-22 is an automatic microprocessor controlled reprocessing system capable of handling up to four dialyzers simultaneously. The reuse procedure performed by the system consists of a bidirectional water flush of the blood compartment, a reverse ultrafiltration with a transmembrane pressure of 850–900 mmHg, followed by a second water flush lasting 5, 15, and 5 min, respectively. This is followed by a hydrogen peroxide rinse (0.5%). After completion of the blood compartment rinse, a positive pressure of 600–800 mmHg is induced in the blood compartment with the outlet closed to assure fiber expansion. A measurement of the dialyzer's blood compartment volume is automatically performed, and the operator is warned if volume falls below 80% of the original value. A satisfactory blood compartment volume test is followed by pressure testing in which the blood compartment volume test is followed by pressure testing in which the blood compartment is subjected to a pressure of 250 mmHg while the dialysate compartment is at atmospheric pressure. If the pressure decrease in the blood compartment exceeds 1 mmHg/s, the dialyzer is rejected. Finally, the dialyzers are filled with a formaldehyde solution (3%), removed from the machine, and stored.

REASONS FOR DECLINING UTILIZATION OF REUSE IN THE UNITED KINGDOM

Analysis of the replies to our questionnaire from United Kingdom dialysis centers have highlighted the following four principal reasons for the decline of this practice in recent years: the impact of reuse on the functional performance of the device, concern over formaldehyde exposure to staff and patients when reusing, a variable reuse achievement, and financial considerations. Other reasons cited included inconvenience, time taken for reuse, pressure from patients, and infection. Our experiences relating to the principal reasons cited when using the three reuse techniques described are discussed below.

FUNCTIONAL PERFORMANCE OF HEMODIALYZERS ON REUSE

During dialysis, blood products and protein are deposited on the membrane surface, causing loss of surface area, or obstruction of blood passages, leading to a decreased membrane permeability and loss of efficiency. Adequate removal of these products is desirable to ensure that on subsequent use the dialyzer performs in a manner comparable with that on first use.

Traditionally, when nondisposable dialyzers were used, each dialyzer was used three times so that it needed rebuilding only once a week. A review of the current United Kingdom reuse practice shows that, on average, six uses

Table 8-4. In vivo urea clearance characteristics at a blood flow of 200 ml/min[a]

Dialyzer	First use	Reuse method	3rd use	4th use	6th use	7th use
MTS Hemoflow	172 ± 2 (16)	Manual	172 ± 2 (11)		167 ± 3 (6)	
Gambro Lundia Fiber	143 ± 2 (12)	Texas ADR22		137 ± 4 (12)		136 ± 6 (12)
Hospal Disscap	133 ± 18 (12)	Texas ADR22		140 ± 13 (12)		141 ± 14 (12)
Hospal Biospal 2400	154 ± 11[b] (8)	ABG Semca	152 ± 13 (6)		179 ± 19 (5)	
Asahi PAN 150	117 ± 12 (12)	Texas ADR22		104 ± 12 (12)		92 ± 12 (12)

[a]Figures in parentheses refer to number of measurements.
[b]Measurements performed using Hospal Monitral system. Mean ± 2 SD shown

Table 8-5. In vivo creatinine clearance characteristics at a blood flow of 200 ml/min[a]

Dialyzer	First use	Reuse method	3rd use	4th use	6th use	7th use
MTS Hemoflow	137 ± 4 (16)	Manual	133 ± 2 (11)		133 ± 5 (6)	
Gambro Lundia Fiber	108 ± 5 (12)	Texas ADR22		100 ± 12 (12)		104 ± 6 (12)
Hospal Disscap	93 ± 20 (12)	Texas ADR22		106 ± 15 (12)		102 ± 9 (12)
Hospal Biospal 2400	119 ± 8[b] (8)	ABG Semca	116 ± 10 (6)		138 ± 16 (5)	
Asahi PAN 150	99 ± 14 (12)	Texas ADR22		89 ± 10 (12)		77 ± 12 (12)

[a]Figures in parentheses refer to number of measurements.
[b]Measurements performed using Hospal Monitral system. Mean ± 2 SD shown.

Table 8-6. Ultrafiltration coefficient[a]

Dialyzer	Reuse method	First use	3rd use	4th use	6th use	7th use
MTS Hemoflow	Manual	3.6 ± 0.6 (34)	3.1 ± 0.9 (21)		3.1 ± 0.6 (11)	
Gambro Lundia Fiber	Texas ADR22	7.1 ± 1.1 (10)		7.1 ± 1.4 (10)		7.7 ± 1.8 (10)
Hospal Disscap	Texas ADR22	7.1 ± 1.2 (10)		6.4 ± 1.2 (10)		7.7 ± 1.8 (10)
Asahi PAN 150	Texas ADR22	61 ± 22.8 (10)		37 ± 18.3 (10)		24.6 ± 17.1 (10)

[a]Mean ± SD shown. Figures in parentheses refer to number of observations.

(first use and five reuses) are attempted for each dialyzer, although some dialysis units aim for as many as nine uses. To assess the influence of reuse on the in vivo functional performance, namely, clearance and ultrafiltration, we studied these parameters in dialyzers with CUPROPHAN® membranes (MTS Hemoflow 1.3 m^2, Gambro Lundia Fibre GF 120H 1.2 m^2, Hospal Disscap 1.4 m^2) and polyacrylonitrile membranes (Hospal Biospal 2400 [AN69S], Asahi PAN 150). The latter were used for hemodiafiltration, when reprocessed by the three techniques described above. Measurements to assess clearance and ultrafiltration were performed during the second hour of treatment. Blood flows were measured by bubble transit techniques [13]. Data have been analyzed by a method of least squares curve fit procedure, with results shown for a blood flow of 200 ml/min in tables 8-4 and 8-5. The ultrafiltration coefficients (ml/h/mmHg) established during first and subsequent use are shown in table 8-6. The ultrafiltration characteristics of the Biospal 2400 were not measured, since the dialyzer was used with the Hospal Monitral single patient system, which offers volumetric ultrafiltration control.

The clearance of small molecules fell slightly on reuse. It is unlikely, however, that the magnitude of the observed changes have any clinical significance. The interpretation of these changes is difficult unless they can be correlated with effective surface area, since any reduction in clearance and ultrafiltration may be a consequence of changes in effective surface area or membrane permeability, the latter assuming increased importance particularly when using sodium hypochlorite to clean the dialyzer.

While the presence of active chlorine is beneficial in cleaning the dialyzer due to its weakening of the bonds of fibrin and white cells that are deposited on the membranes, it also has a tendency to weaken the membrane, thereby limiting the number of times the dialyzer may be used. In our early studies, using sodium hypochlorite to rinse polyacrylonitrile-containing hemodialyzers, we attained an overall leak rate of 1.8%, which was marginally higher than for CUPROPHAN®-containing dialyzers that were not exposed to sodium hypochlorite. The majority of leaks occurred during the fifth and sixth use of the dialyzers [14]. We subsequently altered our procedure by reducing the concentration of sodium hypochlorite to 0.5%, obtained by mixing equal parts of MILTON® (stabilized hypochlorite solution containing 1% [wt/vol] sodium hypochlorite and 16.5% [wt/vol] sodium chlorite) with treated water. While 0.5% hypochlorite eliminated blood leaks, the question remained of whether exposure of membrane to this solution altered membrane characteristics. If so, observed changes in functional performance with reuse may reflect the opposing effects of loss of surface area and an increase in membrane permeability. To assess the possibility that exposure to sodium hypochlorite may alter membrane permeability, we performed a series of experiments in which clearance and ultrafiltration characteristics of the dialyzers were measured before and after exposure to sodium hypochlorite for varying lengths of time (table 8-7).

Table 8-7. Effect of sodium hypochlorite (0.5% wt/vol) exposure on functional performance of a hollow-fiber hemodialyzer (MTS Hemoflow)[a]

	No exposure	24-min exposure	36-min exposure
Urea clearance (ml/min)	183 ± 2.5	181 ± 1.9	182 ± 1.5
Creatinine clearance (ml/min)	156 ± 1.5	152 ± 4.3	153 ± 3.3
Vitamin B12 clearance (ml/min)	46 ± 0.9	43.2 ± 2.8	43.1 ± 1.1
Ultrafiltration coefficient (ml/min)	5.54	5.34	5.36

[a]Number of dialyzers studied = 2.

Table 8-8. Relationship between fiber bundle volume and functional performance

	Use 1	Use 3	Use 6
Creatinine[a] clearance (ml/min)	137 ± 3.8	133 ± 1.8	133 ± 5.3
UF coefficient (ml/h/mmHg)	3.6	3.1	3.1
Fiber bundle[b] volume (ml)	78 ± 10	68 ± 10	66 ± 15[c]
Number of measurements	14	11	7

[a]Mean ± 2 SD.
[b]Mean ± SD.
[c]Measured after use 5.

Techniques of measurement of effective surface area in flat-plate hemodialyzers are complex and unsuitable for routine use. In the case of hollow-fiber hemodialyzers, the effective membrane area of the dialyzer is directly related to the fiber bundle volume, and this parameter is widely used as an index of prediction to assess the dialyzer's suitability for further use. In table 8-8, the changes in functional performance (creatinine clearance and ultrafiltration coefficient) have been correlated with fiber bundle volume after six uses. The average fiber bundle volume decrease of 15% correlated well with membrane permeability changes (14%), but poorly with the clearance of small molecules. See chapter 3 for a detailed discussion of this issue.

FORMALIN

Formaldehyde (CH_2O) reacts with the amino groups of proteins and amino acids. For this reason it is used widely as a sterilant. In hemodialysis units it is used for sterilizing equipment such as dialysate delivery or proportionating systems and water purification equipment as well as dialyzers. The use of formaldehyde as a sterilant for hemodialyzers was first described by Pollard et al. [15]. Its use poses risks not only to patients but also to staff since occupational exposure to formaldehyde may be associated with respiratory tract and eye irritation. A spillage of 1 ml of 37% formalin in a 3 × 4 × 7-m room will, if completely volatized, produce vapors about 3.6 ppm. Formaldehyde at levels above 0.13 ppm is known to be an irritant in occupational settings and the threshold limit value for acute exposure is 2 ppm. Prolonged handling of formaldehyde by staff and patients is associated with contact dermatitis and asthma [16−18].

A more serious concern is its carcinogenicity or cocarcinogenicity. Animals exposed to atmospheric levels of 6 and 15 ppm over and 18-month period have developed nasal squamous cell carcinomas. A recent epidemiologic survey in humans having long-term exposure to formaldehyde in the chemical industry does not support the animal findings, but the authors of the survey state that the strength of negative evidence is diminished by the small number (605) of subjects exposed to high levels of formaldehyde for more than five years and followed more than 20 years after first exposure [19]. Patients undergoing regular dialysis treatment who are rebuilding their own dialyzers, or reusing at home, are subject to the same risks unless adequate precautions are taken to minimize formaldehyde exposure. Another potential hazard is that in patients receiving regular dialysis treatment the increased presence of anti-N-like antibodies has been observed. (See chapter 9 for details.)

MEASUREMENT OF FORMALDEHYDE LEVELS WHEN REUSING

Koch et al. [23] performed a series of measurements to assess the minimum formaldehyde level capable of producing alterations of the red cell membrane that makes the erythrocyte more susceptible to anti-N-like antibodies. They found that such alterations did not occur at formaldehyde levels below 10 μg/ml, while Lewis et al. [24] showed that residual formaldehyde levels below 1 μg/ml were not associated with the formation of anti-N-like antibodies.

Following the recommendation of Pollard et al. [15], the most widely used test for demonstrating the presence of formaldehyde in the dialyzer has been the CLINITEST tablet, a commercially available test system used for the semiquantitative determination of glucose in the urine. The color of the test fluid changes from blue to brown when sufficient amounts of reducing substances are present.

A much more sensitive procedure for the measurement of formaldehyde concentration is Hantzsch reaction, which permits highly specific colorimetric quantitation of as little as 1 µg/ml formaldehyde. For such measurements, equal volumes of acetylacetone reagent (2 mol ammonium acetate, 0.05 mol acetic acid, 0.02 mol acetylacetone added to 1 liter of distilled water) and the formaldehyde-containing sample are mixed. The color developed after 1 h of incubation is measured in a spectrophotometer at 412 nm. Such a method is time consuming and complicated for routine use. For the latter, Schiff's reagent (a solution of fuchine sulphorous acid) may be more suitable. More recently, semiquantitative methods using prepacked reagents have become available (FORMALERT [Organon Teknika, Turnhout, Belgium], FORMOTEST [Hydro-M, Lyon, France]).

To assess the adequacy of CLINITEST tablets, Schiff's reagent, and FORM-ALERT in detecting residual formaldehyde during reuse, we tested a series of solutions containing from 0 to 4500 mg/liter formaldehyde (µg/ml). Table 8-9 summarizes the results obtained with the CLINITEST tablets. Pollard et al. [15], in their original method, used 0.5 ml of test solution mixed with a single CLINITEST tablet. Such a combination failed to detect concentrations of formaldehyde below 90 µg/ml. Furthermore, acetate- and bicarbonate-containing dialysates both gave a positive reaction (due to the dextrose contained within them) as saline which had been dialyzed against a dextrose-containing dialysate for a period of 20 min. To check the sensitivity of the test using differing volumes of test solutions, the studies were repeated with 1 and 5 ml of test solution. The range of 0.5–5 ml represents the extreme ranges of volumes that might be added to the tablet at the bedside if pipettes were not used; 15 s after the boiling reaction had stopped the tube containing the test solution was shaken and the color noted. A negative reaction was indicated by a blue color while the presence of aldehyde was denoted by a green/orange color. The sensitivity of the method did not change when 1 ml of test solution was added, but it diminished considerably if 5 ml of test solution was mixed with the CLINITEST tablet.

When using the Schiff's reagent, the technique is to add 1 ml of reagent to 1 ml of test solution. As with the CLINITEST tablets the studies were repeated with 0.5 and 5 ml of test solutions being added to 1 ml of reagent. When using such combinations, a negative reaction was indicated by clear solution, while a color change to pink or purple denoted the presence of aldehyde (table 8-10). In common with the CLINITEST findings, such a test again gave false-positive results for dialysate.

FORMALERT® is prepackaged in individual ampules containing 0.2 ml of reagent to which the manufacturers specify the addition of 1 ml of formaldehyde-containing solution, the ampule being shaken after the addition of the test fluid and the color reaction observed. The time of reaction varies with the concentration of formaldehyde present. At high concentrations an instant reaction occurs, but at low concentrations the reaction may

Table 8-9. Measurement of residual formaldehyde using CLINITEST tablets[a]

Volume of test solution (ml)	Concentration of formaldehyde (mg/liter)											Dialysate		Saline	
	0	4500	900	450	180	90	45	18	9	4.5	2.25	S509[b]	HCO$_3$[c]	S509[d]	HCO$_3$[e]
0.5	−	+	+	+	+	+	−	−	−	−	−	+	+	+	+
1.0	−	+	+	+	+	+	−	−	−	−	−	+	+	+	+
5.0	−	+	+	−	−	−	−	−	−	−	−	+	−	−	+

[a] +, positive reaction; and −, no reaction.
[b] Renalyte S509 acetate-based concentrate containing 2.0 g/liter dextrose on dilution (1:34).
[c] Renalyte B$_{11}$ bicarbonate-based concentrate containing 2.0 g/liter dextrose on dilution.
[d] Saline from the blood compartment of the dialyzer in which acetate-based dialysate had been used following a 20-min blood flow stagnation period.
[e] Saline from the blood compartment of the dialyzer in which bicarbonate-based dialysate had been used following a 20-min blood flow stagnation period.

Table 8-10. Measurement of residual formaldehyde using Schiff's reagent[a]

Volume of test solution (ml)	Concentration of formaldehyde (mg/liter)											Dialysate		Saline	
	0	4500	900	450	180	90	45	18	9	4.5	2.25	S509[b]	HCO$_3$[c]	S509[d]	HCO$_3$[e]
0.5	−	+	+	+	+	+	−	−	−	−	−	−	−	−	−
1.0	−	+	+	+	+	+	+	−	−	−	−	+	+	+	+
5.0	−	+	+	+	+	+	−	−	−	−	−	+	+	+	+

[a] +, positive reaction; and −, no reaction.
[b] Renalyte S509 acetate-based concentrate containing 2.0 g/liter dextrose on dilution (1:34).
[c] Renalyte B$_{11}$ bicarbonate-based concentrate containing 2.0 g/liter dextrose on dilution.
[d] Saline from the blood compartment of the dialyzer in which acetate-based dialysate had been used following a 20-min blood flow stagnation period.
[e] Saline from the blood compartment of the dialyzer in which bicarbonate-based dialysate had been used following a 20-min blood flow stagnation period.

Table 8-11. Measurement of residual formaldehyde using FORMALERT®[a]

Volume of test solution (ml)	Concentration of formaldehyde (mg/liter)											Dialysate		Saline	
	0	4500	900	450	180	90	45	18	9	4.5	2.25	S509[b]	HCO3[c]	S509[d]	HCO3[e]
0.5	−	+	+	+	+	+	+	+	+	−	−	−	−	−	−
1.0	−	+	+	+	+	+	+	+	+	+	−	−	−	−	−
2.0	−	+	+	+	+	+	+	+	+	−	−	−	−	−	−

[a] +, positive reaction; and −, no reaction.
[b] Renalyte S509 acetate–based concentrate containing 2.0 g/liter dextrose on dilution (1:34).
[c] Renalyte B11 bicarbonate–based concentrate containing 2.0 g/liter dextrose on dilution.
[d] Saline from the blood compartment of the dialyzer in which acetate–based dialysate had been used following a 20-min blood flow stagnation period.
[e] Saline from the blood compartment of the dialyzer in which bicarbonate–based dialysate had been used following a 20-min blood flow stagnation period.

not occur until 3 min have elapsed. In the series of studies shown in table 8-11, color reactions were read at 5 min after the addition of the test solution. As with Schiff's reagent, a negative reaction is denoted by a clear solution while the presence of formaldehyde is denoted by the appearance of purple. This method of detecting formaldehyde was found to be the most sensitive, detecting concentrations as low as 4.5 µg/ml. Furthermore, false positives were not observed with dextrose-containing dialysates. In our studies we found the sensitivity of the method only marginally impaired if less or more than the specified 1 ml of test solution were added.

MINIMIZING RESIDUAL FORMALDEHYDE LEVELS BEFORE NEXT USE

Our procedure for the preparation of dialyzers for subsequent use after storage with formaldehyde is the following: Rinsing of the dialyzers consists of five periods. In period A (0−30 min), the dialysate side is rinsed with tap water or dialysate, while the blood compartment remains clamped. During period B (30−40 min), the blood lines are connected to the dialyzer, followed by period C during which 2 liters of saline are pumped through the blood compartment with the dialysate flowing. In period D, dialysate continues to flow but the blood lines remain clamped, while the patient or nurse inserts the fistula needles, and the patient is prepared for connection to the extracorporeal circuit. In the final period (E), blood flows in the extracorporeal circuit and the displaced saline is either discarded or infused into the patient, depending on clinical requirements. The formaldehyde levels measured during these five phases in the venous line are shown in figure 8-3. It may be seen that, following the clamping period during which the needles were inserted, a diffusion of formalin into the blood compartment from the membrane occurs, the height of the peak representing the maximum concentration of formaldehyde that may enter the patient's blood stream if the saline in the extracorporeal circuit is not discarded but infused immediately after connection of the patient to the extracorporeal circuit. If the saline is partially discarded because of clinical requirements, the amount of formaldehyde entering the patient's circulation is reduced.

A series of experiments carried out by Lewis et al. [25] to investigate the effects of different methods of rinsing proposed a modification of the procedure, such that in period C only 1.5 liters of saline were rinsed through the blood compartment, after which the blood lines were clamped and the dialyzer allowed to stand for a period of 20 min, during wich the fistula needles were inserted. After insertion, a further 500 ml of saline was used to rinse the extracorporeal circuit, after which the patient could be connected to the extracorporeal circuit or, if required, the circuit partially drained. Figure 8-4 shows that this simple modification results in an appreciable lowering of the formaldehyde concentration so that the fluid entering the patient's vein contains below 2 µg/ml of formaldehyde.

Although this modification of the patient connection procedure lowered

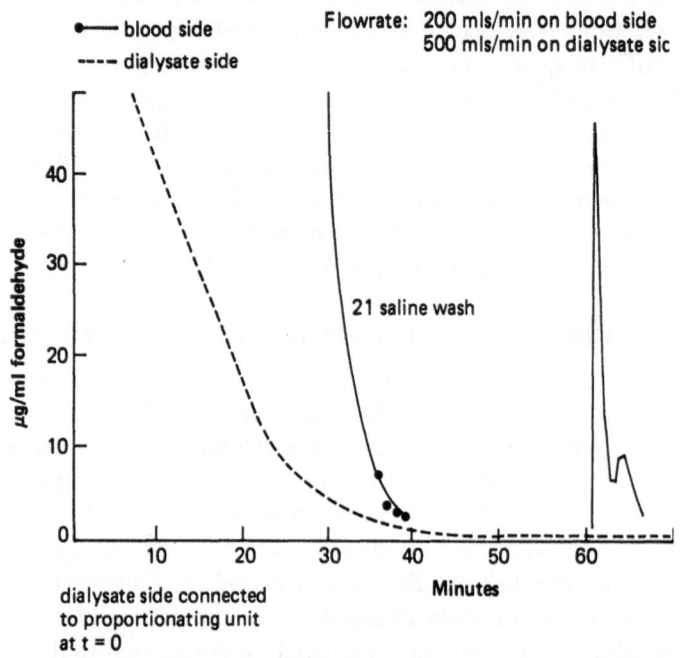

Figure 8-3. Formaldehyde concentration in saline emerging from the venous line of a hollow-fiber hemodialyzer. Reprinted by permission of the International Society for Artificial Organs from Artificial Organs, Volume 5, Number 3, February, 1981. Copyright by the International Society for Artificial Organs.

the level of formaldehyde infused to the patient, formaldehyde remained in the membrane and, when isolated sections of membrane were continuously stirred in a flask, the formaldehyde levels observed continued to rise even after 2 h, suggesting that it is held at least in part in chemical combination by the membrane. (For a discussion of alternate methods for removal of formaldehyde prior to next use, see chapters 2 and 3. The use of recirculation of saline in the blood compartment markedly aids formaldehyde removal.)

The threshold concentration of formaldehyde at which damage to red cells occurs is uncertain. Fassbinder and Koch suggested the critical level to be 10 µg/ml [25], while Orringer and Mattern detected one type of red cell injury at concentrations above 3 µg/ml, but it is not known whether this is relevant to the production of anti-N-like antibodies [27]. Lewis et al. [24] showed that *residual* formaldehyde concentrations below 1 µg/ml were not associated with the presence of anti-N-like antibodies. Consequently, it is reasonable to aim for a concentration of 1–2 µg/ml, the lowest detectable concentration using bed-side techniques.

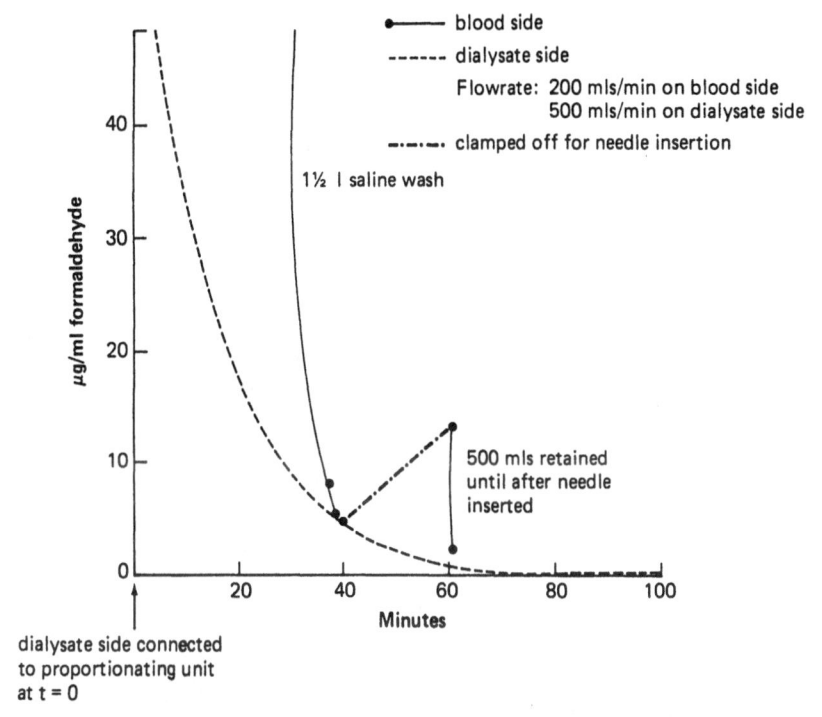

Figure 8-4. Formaldehyde concentration in saline emerging from the venous line of a hollow-fiber hemodialyzer after modification of the blood compartment rinse procedure.

REUSE ACHIEVEMENT

With dialyzers such as the Kiil and the later multipoint variants, the goal was three uses since this meant rebuilding the dialyzer once per week. When reusing disposable dialyzers, many dialysis centers aim for six uses (first use plus five reuses) while some centers aim for a higher number of reuses.

Table 8-12. The role of single and multiple nurse supervision in reuse achievement of hollow-fiber hemodialyzers

	Percentage usage achievement					
	Use 1	2	3	4	5	6
Single nurse supervision	100 (16)[a]	81	69	50	44	38
Multiple nurse supervision	100 (226)[a]	82	59	41	25	11

[a]Number of dialyzers studied.

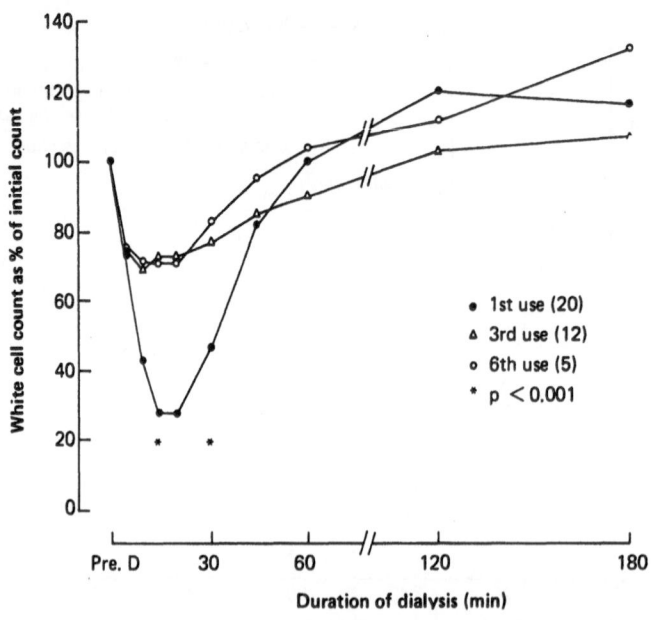

Figure 8-5. Effect of manual reuse technique without chemical exposure on hemodialysis leukopenia. Reprinted with permission of the publisher from Int. J. of Artificial Organs 6:261–266, 1983.

To assess the reality of such aims we have compared the reuse achievement of a single person with that of the dialysis unit staff in general when reusing a hollow-fiber hemodialyzer by manual techniques (table 8-12). For two reuses (corresponding to a single dialyzer per week), single person supervision achieved a 69% success rate compared with a 59% achievement by the dialysis unit staff; in general, by the sixth use (fifth reuse) these differences became more marked.

The most common causes of dialyzer rejection were its cosmetic appearance at the end of dialysis (all dialyzers reused had clear perspex outer casings), or the failure to achieve the required fiber bundle volume, which was set at 90% of the volume of a new dialyzer. Accidental damage to dialyzers during the reuse process and the failure to observe the reuse protocol were the next common causes for dialyzer rejection.

Use of the automated multiple reuse system (Texas Instruments ADR 22), which removes some of the objective bias from the above series, resulted in the discarding of 24 dialyzers (13%) in a group of 187. Of these, 13 were discarded because of failure to achieve the required fiber bundle volume, while in the remaining 11 dialyzers the pressure leak test was positive. The attainment of an average of 5.59 times reuse occurred when using CUPROPHAN®-containing hemodialyzers.

Using the same system on 56 hemodialyzers containing polyacrylonitrile,

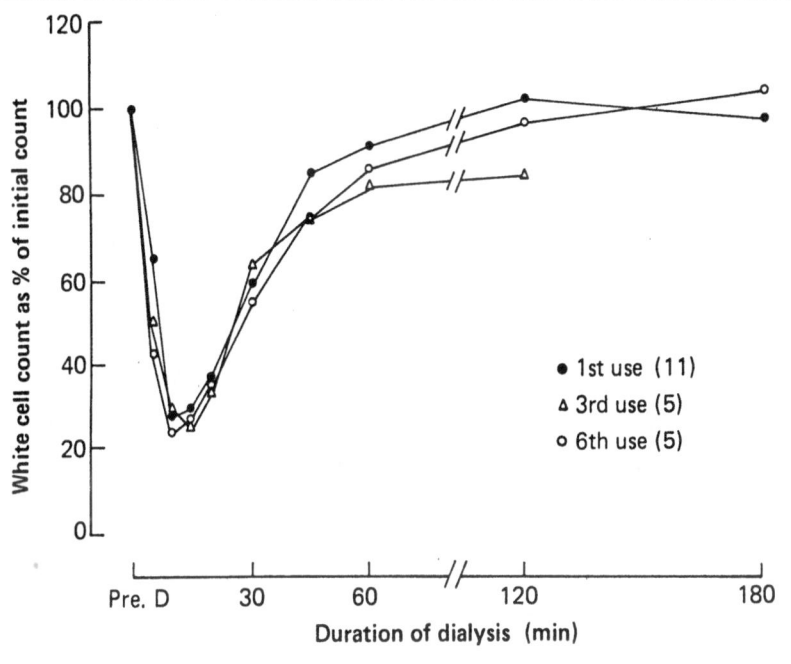

Figure 8-6. Effect of automated reuse technique involving chemical(0.5% sodium hypochlorite) exposure on hemodialysis leukopenia. Reprinted with permission of the publisher from Int. J. of Artificial Organs 6:261–266, 1983.

more than 40% were discarded principally for reasons of volume loss before the sixth reuse. A significant decrease in fiber bundle volume had occurred by the fourth use in 16% of the dialyzers used.

MORBIDITY AND MORTALITY WHEN REUSING

Pyrogen reactions were common in the early days of hemodialysis and were attributed to the reuse of components in direct contact with blood that were sterilized between use.

The mortality and morbidity when reusing has been reviewed by Wing et al. [5] and is discussed in chapter 7.

These reviews as well as other published material on this topic [34, 35] suggest that mortality and morbidity of hemodialysis is improved in patients who are reusing compared with those who are not, possibly due to the elimination of the "new dialyzer syndrome" [36].

POSSIBLE ADVANTAGES OF REUSE

During hemodialysis, changes in white cell counts and complement activation occur [37–40]. We have compared leukopenia on the dialyzer's first use with that on the third and sixth uses when using the manual wash technique, and when exposing the membranes to sodium hypochlorite (figures 8–5 and

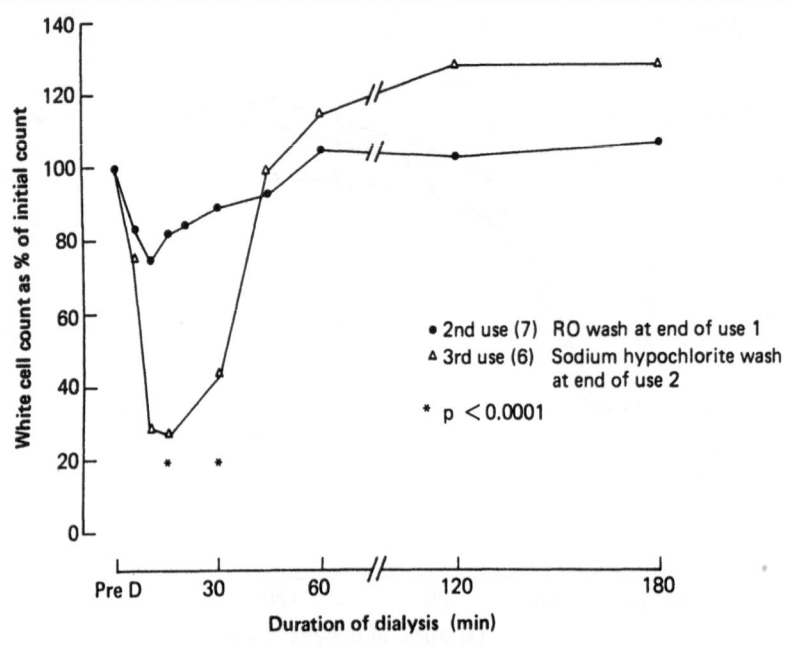

Figure 8-7. The role of sodium hypochlorite in modifying hemodialysis leukopenia observed during reuse. Reprinted with permission of the publisher from Int. J. of Artificial Organs 6:261−266, 1983.

8-6). Falls in white cell count for the dialyzer's first use were comparable for both groups. By the third use, using the manual technique, a significant reduction in the magnitude of leukopenia was noted. Continued reuse, however, failed to promote a further change. In contrast, in the group of dialyzers that were chemically washed, white cell changes remained unaltered even by the sixth use. These differences suggest that the modification of white cell changes observed are a consequence of the deposition of the patient's blood proteins on the membrane surface, which the manual technique of reuse removes partially and which is either totally removed or modified by exposure to sodium hypochlorite. The role of sodium hypochlorite in modifying this phenomenon has been described by Gagon and Kaye [34] and confirmed by our own studies in which the method of membrane cleaning at the termination of dialysis was changed (figure 8-7).

Craddock et al. have proposed that leukopenia observed during hemodialysis is related to complement activation and contributes to hypoxemia [38−40], but this is by no means universally accepted [35, 41, 42].

The effect of hemodialyzer reuse on neutropenia and complement activation is well recognized [43] and has again received renewed interest [44−45]. Our own studies summarized in tables 8-13 and 8-14 partially confirm these findings, notably in terms of C3a, which on reuse is diminished. Observa-

Table 8-13. Complement activation during reuse of CUPROPHAN®-containing hemodialyzers when reusing by a manual technique[a]

Use of dialyzer	Dialysis duration (min)	CH50	Alternative pathway	C3 nephelometry	Factor-B nephelometry	C3a RIA	C3d
First (n = 5)	15	90.2 ± 3.7	103.1 ± 12.1	91.9 ± 4.1	97.0 ± 7.0	632.1 ± 137.6	141.8 ± 21.1
	60	91.7 ± 6.1	97.5 ± 10.5	74.5 ± 10.8	78.7 ± 6.8	615.9 ± 88.9	185.3 ± 32.0
	240	—	93.1 ± 9.7	101.9 ± 6.6	104.6 ± 6.1	198.3 ± 26.2	197.8 ± 13.7
Third (n = 5)	15	97.2 ± 5.1	87.3 ± 9.5	82.9 ± 7.1	80.4 ± 4.6	145.5 ± 63.8	113.1 ± 16.2
	60	99.3 ± 4.6	96.9 ± 4.3	91.1 ± 8.3	92.7 ± 7.8	124.2 ± 26.1	108.3 ± 7.7
Sixth (n = 5)	15	92.8 ± 4.5	113.1 ± 18.0	85.8 ± 2.8	84.4 ± 4.1	150.9 ± 35.7	96.1 ± 16.9
	60	98.9 ± 2.1	102.9 ± 4.6	91.6 ± 2.9	90.8 ± 3.7	103.3 ± 37.8	109.2 ± 6.1

[a]Data (mean ± SEM) expressed as a percentage of predialysis values.

Table 8-14. Complement activation during reuse of CUPROPHAN®-containing hemodialyzers when reusing without and with sodium hypochlorite exposure of the membrane[a]

Use of dialyzer	Dialysis duration (min)	CH50	Alternative pathway	C3 nephelometry	Factor-B nephelometry	C3a RIA	C3d
First (n = 5)	15	90.2 ± 3.7	103.1 ± 12.1	91.9 ± 4.1	97.0 ± 7.0	632.1 ± 137.6	141.8 ± 21.1
	60	91.7 ± 6.1	97.5 ± 10.5	74.5 ± 10.8	78.7 ± 6.8	615.9 ± 88.9	185.3 ± 32.0
Second[1] (n = 5)	15	96.2 ± 2.4	108.9 ± 5.5	94.3 ± 1.2	94.1 ± 2.5	191.4 ± 47.9	107.3 ± 13.4
	60	102.6 ± 0.7	111.3 ± 8.9	101.4 ± 2.1	106.1 ± 1.2	214.9 ± 50.2	110.8 ± 15.3
Third[2] (n = 5)	15	98.2 ± 2.9	91.5 ± 3.9	87.6 ± 4.3	85.4 ± 5.4	470.1 ± 289.4	139.0 ± 18.3
	60	97.0 ± 3.0	88.9 ± 12.7	81.0 ± 6.4	84.6 ± 6.7	1736.0 ± 65.4	148.5 ± 11.5

[a]Data (mean ± SEM) expressed as a percentage of predialysis values.

tions relating to other complement components do not show such clear-cut improvement with reuse, possibly due to the different sensitivities of the methods used to quantify such changes.

In summary, different membranes show differences in their ability to activate complement and induce leukopenia. Dialysis with reused membranes modifies these phenomena, but their clinical implications are far from clear, particularly as the changes induced on reusing cellulose-based membranes are such as to make them comparable with those observed during the first use of synthetic membranes. In a recent paper by Hakim et al. [46], however, an association between the level of complement activation and adverse reactions experienced during hemodialysis has been established and, consequently, these changes and their possible implications require further study. See chapter 10 for an extensive discussion of these factors.

GUIDELINES FOR REUSE

Reuse of hemodialyzers is a controversial practice. The issues surrounding it are complex and involve medical, ethical, social, and financial considerations. Despite these complex issues, it remains firmly established.

Manufacturers of disposable hemodialyzers produce products that are sterile, safe, effective, and offer a high degree of reliability because of the rigid quality control procedures imposed during their production. In addition, manufacturers of devices are subject to inspection by regulatory authorities to ensure that they meet Good Manufacturing Practice (GMP) requirements.

No dialysis center is subject to such rigorous control or legislation and, consequently, the need for correct and strictly programmed procedures at every stage of the reuse process cannot be over emphasized.

Currently, no national codes of practice exist in the United Kingdom or in Europe relating to reuse of devices intended for single use although some centers have drawn up their own guidelines. (The reader is referred to chapter 12, where the status of the development of a recommended practice for reuse of hemodialyzers in the United States is discussed.)

It is our belief that potential or existing proponents of this practice should address themselves to the following:

1. Can the hemodialyzer be adequately cleaned at the termination of treatment in order to permit reuse?
2. Can the device be processed for reuse without changing the quality of treatment offered and, if so, at what point does the quality of treatment begin to change adversely?
3. Is the resterilization process effective and can the sterilant be effectively removed from the device?

In addition to these fundamental issues, prospective and existing reusers should also ensure that all water used for reprocessing is of an adequate bacteriologic standard. A system of accurate records is kept for reuse in which clinical morbidity is accurately recorded and the basis for rejection of each dialyzer is indicated, and the techniques employed utilize a marking system that uniquely and simply identifies each patient. Staff or patients reusing should also be offered adequate environmental protection against the adverse effects of formaldehyde. It must be recognized that the practice of reuse may not be in the clinical interest of every patient and that routine monitoring for the presence of anti-N-like antibodies is performed in those patients who are reusing.

ACKNOWLEDGMENTS

We should like to express our appreciation to colleagues at Newcastle upon Tyne (C. Woffindin, D. Levett, S.R.D. Johnson, P. Buckley, J. Harden, C. Jack, and K. Fletcher) and Gent (R. van Holder, M. Piron, R. Veirman, A. de Cubber, and N. Vermaercke) for their contributions to the studies described.

REFERENCES

1. Pendras JP, Cole JJ, Tu WH, Scribner BH: Improved technique of continuous flow hemodialysis. Trans Am Soc Artif Intern Organs 7:27–36, 1961.
2. Von Hartitzsch B, Hoenich NA: Meltec multipoint haemodialyser. Br Med J 1:237–239, 1972.
3. Shaldon S, Silva H, Rosen SM: Technique of refrigerated coil preservation haemodialysis with femoral venous catheterization. Br Med J 2:411–413, 1964.
4. Wing AJ, Broyer M, Brunner FP, et al: Combined reports on regular dialysis and transplantation in Europe. XIII. Proc Eur Dial Transplant Assoc 20:2–75, 1983.
5. Wing AJ, Brunner FP, Brynger HOA, et al.: Mortality and morbidity of reusing dialysers. Br Med J 2:853–855, 1978.
6. Deane N, Bemis JA: Multiple use of hemodialyzers. In: Drukker W, Parsons FM, Maher JF (eds) Replacement of renal function by dialysis. Martinus Nijhoff, Boston, 1983, pp 286–304.
7. Hakim RM: Evaluation of the efficacy and safety of SPORICIDIN-HD for disinfecting new and reused dialyzers and hemodialysis machines. Dial Transplant 13:769–778, 1984.
8. Craske H, Dabrowiecki M, Kennedy I, et al.: Evaluation of dialyzer reuse at Toronto Western Hospital. Artif Organs 6:208–213, 1982.
9. Fitzcharles N, Elliot HL, Macdougall AI: Clinical evaluation of an automated system for dialyzer reuse. Dial Transplant 9:825–828, 1980.
10. Hardy DW, Higgins MR, McFarlane DF, Hughes RV: An automated cleaning device for dialyzers: machine design and technology. Clin Nephrol 5:275–278, 1976.
11. De Palma JR, Mason B, Abukurah AR: New artificial kidney reuse machine. Trans Am Soc Artif Intern Organs 20:584–588, 1974.
12. Man NK, Glace M, Becker A, Di Giulio S, Zingraff J, Funck-Brentano JL: A new dialyzer re-use machine. In: Conference on technical aspects of renal dialysis. Newcastle upon Tyne, 1978, pp 73–79.
13. Hoenich NA, Kerr DNS: Dialysers. In: Drukker W, Parsons FM, Maher JF (eds) Replacement of renal function by dialysis. Martinus Nijhoff, Boston, 1983, pp 106–141.
14. Hoenich NA, Kerr DNS, Ward MK, Aljama P, Sussman M: Two special properties of polyacrylonitrile membrane: suitability for reuse and biocompatibility. Contemp Dial 5(1):31–41, 1984.
15. Pollard TL, Barnett BMS, Eschbach JW, Scribner BH: A technique for storage and multiple re-use of the Kiil dialyzer and blood tubing. Trans Am Soc Artif Intern Organs 13:24–28, 1967.

16. Sakula A: Formalin asthma in hospital laboratory staff. Lancet 2:816, 1975.
17. Porter JAH: Acute respiratory distress following formalin inhalation. Lancet 2:603–604, 1975.
18. Hendrick DJ, Lane DJ: Formalin asthma in hospital staff. Br Med J 1:607–608, 1975.
19. Acheson ED, Gardner MJ, Pannett B, Barnes HRR, Osmond C, Taylor CP: Formaldehyde in the British chemical industry. Lancet 1:611–616, 1984.
20. Fassbinder W, Seidl S, Koch KM: The role of formaldehyde in the formation of haemodialysis-associated anti-N-like antibodies. Vox Sang 35:41–48, 1978.
21. Kaehny WD, Miller GE, White WL: Relationship between dialyzer reuse and the presence of anti-N-like antibodies in chronic hemodialysis patients. Kidney Int 12:59–65, 1977.
22. Sandler SG, Sharon R, Bush M, Stroup M, Sabo B: Formaldehyde-related antibodies in hemodialysis patients. Transfusion 19:682–687, 1978.
23. Koch KM, Frei U, Fassbinder W: Hemolysis and anemia in anti-N-like antibody positive hemodialysis patients. Trans Am Soc Artif Intern Organs 24:709–713, 1978.
24. Lewis KJ, Dewar PJ, Ward MK, Kerr DNS: Formation of anti-N-like antibodies in dialysis patients: effect of different methods of dialyzer rinsing to remove formaldehyde. Clin Nephrol 15:39–43, 1981.
25. Lewis KJ, Ward MK, Kerr DNS: Residual formaldehyde in dialyzers: quantity, location and the effect of different methods of rinsing. Artif Organs 5:269–277, 1981.
26. Fassbinder W, Koch KM: A specific immunohaemolytic anaemia induced by formaldehyde sterilisation of dialysers. Contrib Nephrol 36:51–67, 1983.
27. Orringer EP, Mattern WD: Formaldehyde-induced hemolysis during chronic hemodialysis. N Engl J Med 294:1416–1420, 1976.
28. Foxen LG: Is reuse cost effective? A case study. Dial Transplant 13:290–293, 1984.
29. Matthew TH, Fazzalari RA, Disney APS, MacIntyre DB: Multiple use of dialyzers: an Australian view. Nephron 27:222–225, 1981.
30. Leuhmann D, Hirsch D, Carlson G, Constantini E, Keshaviah P: Dialyzer reuse in a large dialysis program. Trans Am Soc Artif Intern Organs 28:76–80, 1982.
31. Siemsen A, Coad RJ, Wong EGC, Sugihara JG, Musgrave JE, Basilio R: Economic impact of an integrated approach to hemodialysis and dialyzer reuse. Dial Transplant 9:933–936, 1980.
32. Deane N, Blagg C, Bower J, et al.: A survey of dialyzer reuse practice in the United States. Dial Transplant 7:1128–1130, 1978.
33. Kant KS, Pollak VE, Cathey M, Goetz D, Berlin R: Multiple use of dialyzers: safety and efficacy. Kidney Int 19:728–738, 1981.
34. Gagnon RF, Kaye M: Hemodialysis neutropenia and dialyzer reuse: role of the cleansing agent. Uremia Invest 8:17–23, 1984.
35. Aljama P, Bird PAE, Ward MK, et al.: Haemodialysis-induced leucopenia and activation of complement: effect of different membranes. Proc Eur Dial Transplant Assoc 15:144–153, 1978.
36. Odgen DA: New-dialyzer syndrome. N Engl J Med 302:1262–1263, 1980.
37. Kaplow LS, Goffinet JA: Profound neutropenia during the early phase of hemodialysis. JAMA 203:133–135, 1968.
38. Craddock PR, Hammerschmidt D, White JG, Dalmasso AP, Jacob HS: Complement (C5a)-induced granulocyte aggregation in vitro. J Clin Invest 60:260–264, 1977.
39. Craddock PR, Fehr J, Brigham KL, Kronenberg RS, Jacob HS: Complement and leukocyte-mediated pulmonary dysfunction in hemodialysis. N Engl J Med 296:769–774, 1977.
40. Craddock PR, Fehr J, Dalmasso AP, Brigham KL, Jacob HS: Hemodialysis leukopenia. J Clin Invest 59:879–888, 1977.
41. Jacob AI, Gavellas G, Zarco R, Perez G, Bourgoignie JJ: Leukopenia, hypoxia and complement function with different hemodialysis membranes. Kidney Int 18:505–509, 1980.
42. Habte B, Carter R, Shamebo M, Veicht J, Boulton Jones JM: Dialysis induced hypoxemia. Clin Nephrol 18:120–125, 1982.
43. Hakim RM, Lowrie EG: Effect of dialyzer reuse on leukopenia, hypoxemia and total hemolytic complement system. Trans Am Soc Artif Intern Organs 26:159–164, 1980.
44. Stroncek DF, Keshaviah P, Craddock PR, Hammerschmidt DE: Effect of dialyzer reuse on complement activation and neutropenia in hemodialysis. J Lab Clin Med 104:304–311, 1984.

45. Chenoweth DE: Biocompatibility of hemodialysis membranes. Am Soc Artif Intern Organ J 7:44−49, 1984.
46. Hakim RM, Breillatt J, Lazarus M, Port FK: Complement activation and hypersensitivity reactions to dialysis membranes. N Engl J Med 311:878−882, 1984.

9. IMMUNE RESPONSE TO REUSE: ANTI-N-LIKE ANTIBODIES

W. FASSBINDER
KARL M. KOCH

In 1972, Howell and Perkins [1] reported a cold agglutinin with apparent anti-N specificity in 12 patients on regular hemodialysis treatment. They termed the new found antibody "anti-N-like" and discussed the possibility that reuse of the dialyzer and its sterilization with formaldehyde might result in the formation of antibodies cross-reacting with the N-receptor of the red cells.

This concept was supported by Harrison et al. [2], who found antibodies with anti-N specificity in the sera of only those hemodialysis patients who reused their dialyzers. To determine whether dialyzer reuse or formaldehyde sterilization are causative factors in the development of anti-N-like antibodies in hemodialysis patients, we screened the sera of 270 hemodialysis patients for cold agglutinins [3]. The serologic methods are described in detail elsewhere [4].

SEROLOGIC CHARACTERIZATION OF ANTI-N-LIKE ANTIBODIES

In 60 of the 270 sera, an antibody (having the characteristics of an anti-N) was detected. It behaved like a cold agglutinin and, with cells of the same MN blood group, gave stronger reactions at lower temperatures. It showed a prominent dosage effect and reacted more strongly with homozygous NN cells than with heterozygous MN cells. MM cells gave negative reactions unless the serum titer with NN cells exceeded 1:16. Patients' autologous cells reacted like homologous donor cells with the same MN typing. Table 9-1

Deane, Wineman, and Bemis (eds.): GUIDE TO REPROCESSING OF HEMODIALYZERS.
© 1986. Martinus Nijhoff Publishing. All rights reserved.

Table 9-1. Agglutination profiles of three anti-N-like-positive sera

Patient	Sex	Blood group	Transfusions	Titer with 0 NN cells at 4°C	Temperatures	Donor cell			Auto
						NN	MN	MM	
P.S.	Female	O, NN	Polytransfused	1:18	37°C	−	−	−	−
					22°C	++	+	−	++
					4°C	+++	++	−	+++
S.D.	Male	B, MN	None	1:32	37°C	++	+	−	+
					22°C	+++	++	−	++
					4°C	++++	+++	+	+++
R.M.	Male	A, MM	None	1:128	37°C	++++	++	−	−
					22°C	++++	++++	++	++
					4°C	++++	++++	++++	++++

Table 9-2. Distribution of blood group phenotypes MM, NN, and MN in all patients and in anti-N-like antibody-positive patients

	Blood group		
	MM	MN	NN
All patients (n = 270)	28%	50%	22%
Antibody-positive patients (n = 60)	25%	53%	22%

Table 9-3. The influence of pretreatment of MM cells with formaldehyde on the agglutination by anti-N-like antibody

	Pretreatment formaldehyde concentration			
Antibody	0%	0.1%	0.4%	1%
Anti-N-like	−	+	++	+++
Anti-N⁻	−	−	−	−
Anti-M	++++	++++	++++	++++
Negative patient's serum	−	−	−	−

Reproduced, with permission, from *Proceedings EDTA* 13:336.

shows typical agglutination profiles of three anti-N-like-positve sera.

Blood transfusions and pregnancies did not play a role in the formation of the antibody, as we found 18 never-transfused male patients with positive sera. There was no relation between the occurrence of the anti-N-like antibody and the patient's own MN blood group (table 9-2). The distribution of the phenotypes MN, NN, and MM in all patients and in the antibody-positive patients was nearly identical.

Further studies were performed to examine the influence of formaldehyde on the agglutinability of the red cells. Erythrocytes were incubated at room temperature for 1 h in isotonic saline containing 0, 0.1%, 0.4%, and 1.0% formaldehyde. The formalinized cells were washed and incubated thereafter at room temperature with five sera containing anti-N-like antibodies (table 9-3). Rising formaldehyde concentration in the preincubation period led to a significantly increased agglutinability of the red cells by the anti-N-like antibodies. Formaldehyde pretreatment did not alter the reactivity with commercially available anti-N or anti-M sera and did not induce nonspecific agglutinability of the red cells, as negative control sera gave consistently negative results. These findings suggest that formaldehyde changes the antigenicity of the red cell membrane, resulting in the creation of a neoantigen,

Table 9-4. Development of an anti-N-like antibody in a dialysis patient

Months of dialysis	Donor cell				
	Untreated			Formalinized (1%)	
	MM	MN	NN	MM	NN
0	−	−	−	−	−
2	−	−	−	−	−
4	−	−	−	−	−
6	−	−	−	+	++
8	−	−	−	++	++
10	−	−	+	++	+++
12	−	+	++	++	+++
15	−	++	+++	++	+++

Patient E.H.; female; 54 years; no blood transfusions; reuse of a formaldehyde-sterilized dialyzer agglutinations read at 22°C.

which induces formation of antibodies cross-reacting with N.

The results of these in vitro studies agree with our observation that the reaction with native NN cells was always preceded by an agglutination of formaldehyde-pretreated cells in patients who produced anti-N-like antibodies during the course of dialysis treatment. Table 9-4 shows the development of an anti-N-like antibody in a dialysis patient using a formaldehyde-sterilized dialyzer. The antibody was first seen in the sixth month. Initially it reacted only with the formaldehyde-pretreated cells, but four months later it reacted with native NN cells as well.

RELATIONSHIP TO REUSE

The incidence of anti-N-like antibodies was clearly related to the use of formaldehyde as dialyzer sterilant (table 9-5). In none of the 74 patients with single use of a nonformaldehyde-sterilized dialyzer could this antibody be detected, whereas ten (28%) of 36 patients with single use and 50 (31%) of 150 patients with reuse of formaldehyde-sterilized dialyzers were postive. The difference between the groups using formaldehyde is not significant. When both groups using formaldehyde are compared with the nonformaldehyde group, the difference is significant by chi-square test ($p<0.005$) in each case.

MECHANISMS OF FORMATION

Our results confirmed the observation of Howell and Perkins, who first described a high incidence of a specific cold agglutinin cross-reacting with anti-N in hemodialysis patients [1]. In accordance with their results, blood transfusions and/or pregnancies as a cause for isoimmunization could be excluded [1]. The development of the antibody was dependent on the duration of the regular hemodialysis treatment. During the first six months of

Table 9-5. Occurrence of anti-N-like antibody with varying dialysis techniques

No reuse No formaldehyde sterilization of dialyzer	0 of 74 patients = 0%	$\left.\begin{array}{l}\\\\\end{array}\right\}$ $\text{chi}^2 = 22.6$ $p < 0.005$
No reuse Formaldehyde sterilization of dialyzer	10 of 36 patients = 28%	$\left.\begin{array}{l}\\\\\end{array}\right\}$ $\text{chi}^2 = 0.2$ NS
Reuse Formaldehyde sterilization of dialyzer	50 of 160 patients = 31%	$\text{chi}^2 = 29.4$ $p < 0.005$

treatment, we never found a patient who was anti-N-like positive. Howell and Perkins [1] discussed (a) the use of cellulose membranes for dialysis, (b) the reuse of the dialyzer, and (c) the use of formaldehyde as a sterilant as possible factors involved in the formation of the anti-N-like antibody. As all patients investigated in our study were dialyzed on cellulose membranes (CUPROPHAN®) and the reuse per se had no influence on the frequency of positive antibody titers, these two factors can be excluded. Our results demonstrate clearly, however, that the use of formaldehyde as a sterilant for the dialyzer plays a role in the formation of the antibody.

Having entered the bloodstream, formaldehyde might alter the red cell membrane sufficiently to render it immunogenic. This concept is supported by our in vitro experiments demonstrating that formaldehyde pretreatment of red cells augmented their agglutinability by the anti-N-like antibodies significantly, and by our observation in longitudinal studies that the anti-N-like antibody reacts first with formalinized cells, and only some time later with untreated cells (see table 9-4).

Probably, formaldehyde interacts with the MN receptor of the red cells, as neuraminidase destroys the receptor of anti-N- and anti-M- as well as the receptor for anti-N-like antibodies [7]. The nature of this chemical reaction is most likely a reduction of a carbohydrate or another substance in the MN receptor, since other aldehydes (glyceraldehyde, acetaldehyde), also reacting as reducing agents, induced a similar modification of the red cell membrane [7]. The finding that formaldehyde pretreatment of the red cells only increased their reaction with the anti-N-like antibodies derived from dialysis patients, whereas the reactivity of the heterologous anti-N remained unchanged (see table 9-3), substantiates the fact that the two antibodies are directed against two related, but slightly different, receptors.

FORMALDEHYDE EXPOSURE OF HEMODIALYSIS PATIENTS

From our observation that hemodialysis patients who never reused their formaldehyde-sterilized dialyzers also develop anti-N-like antibodies, it had to be concluded that, during a routine dialysis with a formaldehyde-sterilized dialyzer, sufficient amounts of formaldehyde enter the patient to render the red cells immunogenic. This result occurred in spite of consistently negative tests with CLINITEST® tablets as recommended by Pollard et al. [5] as the accepted test for demonstration of residual formaldehyde in the dialyzer.

The CLINITEST® tablet test is a commercially available test system for the semiquantitative determination of glucose in the urine. The color of a test fluid is changed from blue to brown when sufficient amounts of reducing substances are in the fluid.

To reevaluate the sensitivity of the CLINITEST® tablet test for formaldehyde, we dissolved a tablet in fluids with known formaldehyde concentrations (0, 20, 50, 100, 500, and 1,000 mg/dl formaldehyde in 0.9% NaCl). When a test fluid volume of 1 ml was added, 100 mg/dl was the lowest concentration

Table 9-6. Formaldehyde concentration in venous effluent of Kiil dialyzers at start of dialysis

Formaldehyde concentration (mg/dl)	No. of observations	Percentage
< 1.0	116	52.7
1.0–9.9	73	33.2
10.0–99.9	30	13.6
> 100.0	1	0.5
Total	220	100.0

found to be positive, and when 2 ml were added, which may easily happen when the test is performed as a bedside screening, 500 mg/dl was the lowest formaldehyde concentration that gave a positive result. From these experiments it became evident that the CLINITEST® tablet test is a very crude method of preventing formaldehyde exposure of the patient.

To measure residual formaldehyde concentration, the sensitive Hantzsch reaction [6], which permits highly specific colorimetric quantitation of as little as 0.01 mg/dl formaldehyde, was used. Equal volumes (2 ml) of acetylacetone reagent (1 mol ammonium acetate, 0.05 mol acetic acid, 0.02 mol acetylacetone added to 1 liter of distilled water) and of the possibly formaldehyde-contaminated fluid were mixed in a tube and incubated for 1 h at 37°C. The color that developed was measured in a spectrophotometer at 412 nm.

When we measured the residual formaldehyde concentration in the venous effluent of 220 Kiil dialyzers routinely prepared for dialysis (Table 9-6), in only 52.7% of the cases did we find concentrations below 1 mg/dl. Even though all of these dialyzers showed a negative reaction with CLINITEST® tablets, in 13.6% of the cases formaldehyde concentrations in the venous effluent exceeded 10 mg/100 ml and in one observation even 100 mg/100 ml. In none of these dialyses did clinical symptoms attributable to formaldehyde toxicity occur.

To compare residual formaldehyde concentrations of different dialyzer types, we standardized the rinsing procedure as follows: the dialysate compartment was rinsed with 500 ml/min dialysate and the blood compartment, starting 15 min later, with 200 ml/min sterile saline. From the venous effluent, specimens were taken when 400 ml saline had passed the dialyzer and thereafter whenever a further 200 ml had passed up to a total rinsing volume of 2000 ml.

Figure 9-1 shows that the mean residual formaldehyde concentration decreases with rinsing volumes. When 1200 ml saline have passed the dialyzer, further changes of formaldehyde concentrations are rather small. When the rinsing procedure is finished, only Kiil dialyzers show a mean residual formaldehyde concentration of much less than 1 mg/dl. Both disposable dialyzers tested (Gambro Optima and CDAK IV) exhibit significantly higher

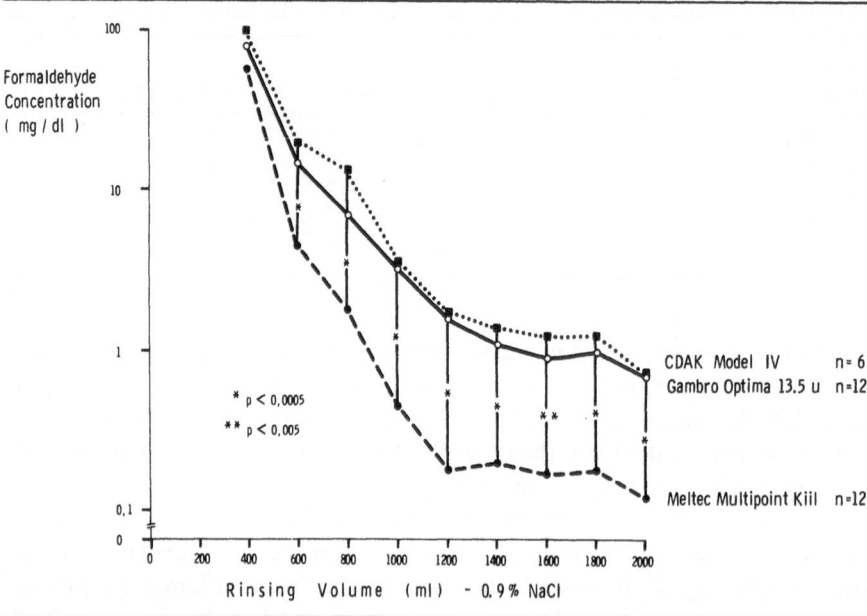

Figure 9-1. Mean residual formaldehyde concentration in three different types of dialyzers. Statistics: Student's *t*-test.

residual formaldehyde concentrations—in the range of 1 mg/dl. A mean formaldehyde concentration in the range of 0.1 mg/dl with a disposable dialyzer of this type was reached only after the first passage of 1000 ml sterile saline, and fluid recirculation in the blood compartment for 30 min; that is, when the formaldehyde was washed out by diffusion into the dialysate compartment which was being rinsed at the same time with 500 ml/min dialysate.

In a further experiment we compared two plate dialyzers (Kiil and Gambro) before first and third use to determine whether reuse would influence the residual formaldehyde concentrations (figure 9-2). In both dialyzer types tested, formaldehyde concentrations did not differ significantly when the first and third uses were compared, but again the mean values of the Kiil dialyzers were significantly lower than those of the disposable dialyzers.

In all these experiments, surprisingly high residual formaldehyde concentrations were found in spite of large rinsing volumes. Obviously, it was impossible by the technique used to render a dialyzer completely free of formaldehyde within an acceptable period of time. This finding suggests that formaldehyde binds to some extent to plastic material or dialyzer membranes during the sterilization phase and dissociates slowly from this binding during the washout phase. On the other hand, it is possible to obtain residual formaldehyde concentrations, which are consistently below a critical threshold of 1.0 mg/dl, when other careful rinsing techniques are applied.

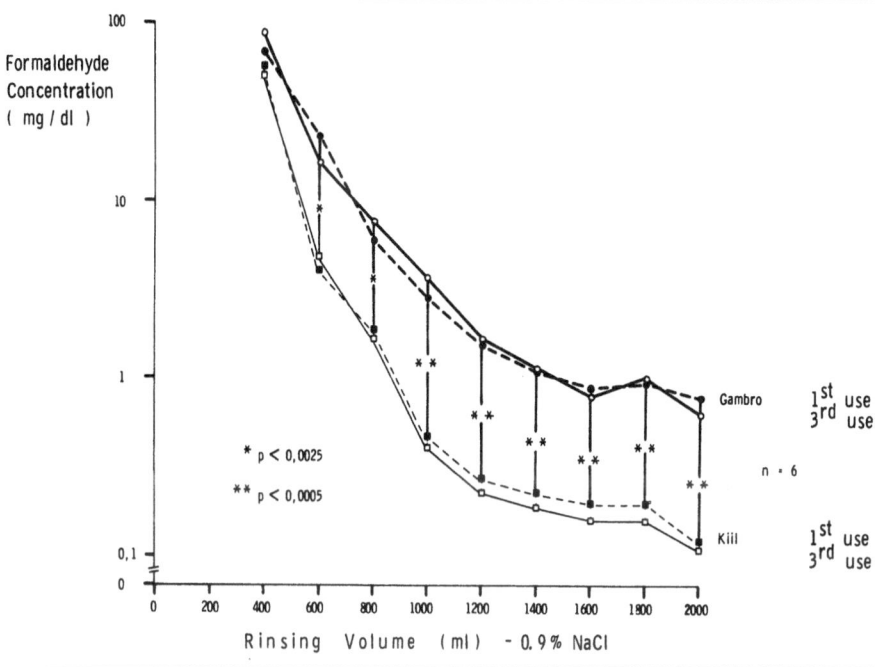

Figure 9-2. Mean residual formaldehyde concentration in a Kiil dialyzer and a disposable plate dialyzer before first and third use. Statistics: Student's *t*-test.

CLINICAL IMPLICATIONS

The development of the hemodialysis-associated anti-N-like antibody has practical consequences: difficulties in blood grouping and cross-matching in patients with anti-N with a high thermal amplitude [7] and failures of renal allografts due to anti-N [8] have been reported. It is therefore recommended that dialysis patients using formaldehyde as sterilant be investigated for the occurrence of these antibodies, especially if they are candidates for renal transplantation.

As anti-N had been described in apparently healthy blood donors [9–12] and in patients with acute autoimmunohemolytic anemia [13–16], we wanted to investigate whether anti-N-like antibodies would cause hemolysis and, if so, whether this hemolysis would contribute to the degree of anemia of hemodialysis patients.

The first investigations were carried out in 27 anti-N-like antibody-positive and 23 anti-N-like antibody-negative patients. All patients were dialyzed on Meltec multipoint 1.0-m² Kiil dialyzers with 11 μm CUPROPHAN® membranes for three times 6–8 h/week. The dialyzers were reused 2–3 times and sterilized with 2% formaldehyde. All patients investigated had been on regular dialysis treatment for at least 25 months. No patient received blood transfusions. The residual formaldehyde concentrations at the start of

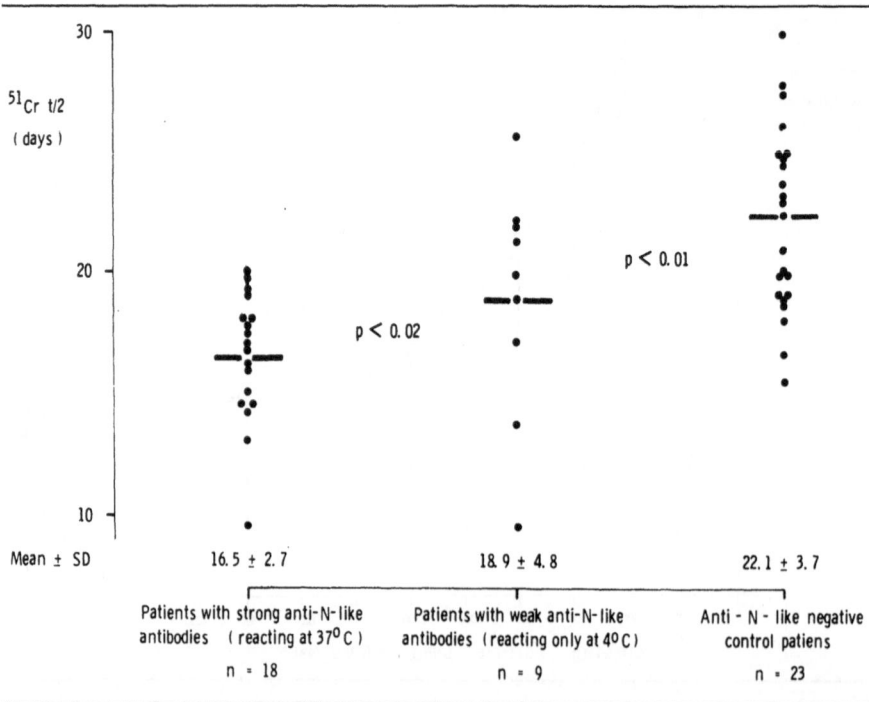

Figure 9-3. [51]Cr half-life of autologous red cells of dialysis patients reusing a formaldehyde-sterilized Kiil dialyzer. Statistics: Student's *t*-test. Reproduced, with permission, from *Trans Am Soc Artif Intern Organs* 24:709−712, 1978.

dialysis were similar to those shown in table 9-6. Red cell half-life (RBC $t\frac{1}{2}$) using standard ^{51}Cr techniques [17] was measured in all patients.

Figure 9-3 shows the results of RBC $t\frac{1}{2}$ measurements during Kiil dialysis. Red cell half-life is expressed as [51]Cr $t/2$. Antibody-positive patients are subdivided into groups having strongly and weakly positive sera. Classification was performed in relation to antibody titer and reaction with NN erythrocytes at 4° and 37°C. Strong sera had titers of 1:16 or more at 4°C and showed a positive reaction at 37°C. The mean (±SD) [51]Cr $t/2$ of patients with strong positive sera was 16.5 ± 2.7 days and significantly ($p < 0.02$) shorter than that of 18.9 ± 4.8 days found in patients with weak positive sera. Antibody-negative control patients exhibited the longest red cell survival, a quarter of them reaching the lower limit of the normal half-life of 25−35 days. The mean [51]Cr $t/2$ in this group was 22.1 ± 3.7 days.

To determine whether formaldehyde and/or reuse contributed to the observed shortening of erythrocyte survival in antibody-positive patients, RBC $t\frac{1}{2}$ was determined again in 12 antibody-positive patients immediately after they had been switched from the reuse of Kiil dialyzers to single use (three times 6−8 h/week) of an ethylene-oxide-sterilized Gambro Optima (1

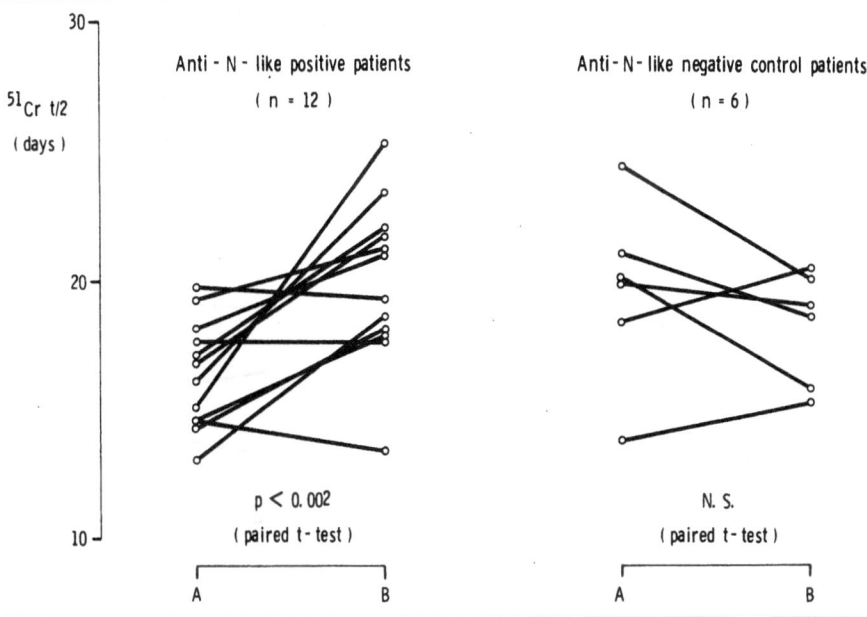

Figure 9-4. ^{51}Cr half-life of autologous red cells during reuse of formaldehyde-sterilized Kiil dialyzers (A) and subsequent single use of ethylene-oxide-sterilized disposable dialyzers (B). Reproduced, with permission, from *Trans Am Soc Artif Intern Organs* 24:709–712, 1978.

m^2, 13.5 μm CUPROPHAN® membrane) disposable dialyzer. Six antibody-negative patients served as controls.

Figure 9-4 shows the comparison of ^{51}Cr $t/2$ measured during reuse of formaldehyde-sterilized Kiil dialyzers and during single use of the ethylene-oxide-sterilized disposable dialyzers. The change of dialyzer and sterilant resulted in a significant ($p < 0.002$, paired t-test) improvement of red cell half-life only in antibody-positive patients, not in antibody-negative controls.

As the ^{51}Cr studies offered an improvement of renal anemia due to reduced hemolysis in antibody-positive patients when formaldehyde sterilization was avoided, these patients were kept on the ethylene-oxide-sterilized dialyzers. Figure 9-5 shows the effect of formaldehyde avoidance on hematocrit in these patients. Hematocrits shown are the mean values of the last four estimations during each treatment period. Time of treatment with ethylene-oxide-sterilized dialyzers ranged from six to 14 months. In the antibody-positive patients the mean hematocrit (±SD) rose from 27.1 ± 3.9 to 30.2 ± 4.2 vol%, whereas in none of the antibody-negative patients was a substantial change documented. The increase of hematocrit in the antibody-positive patients is significant ($p < 0.01$, paired t-test).

As demonstrated in figure 9-6, antibody titers decreased only slowly when the use of formaldehyde was stopped. During the first 3–4 weeks of Gambro

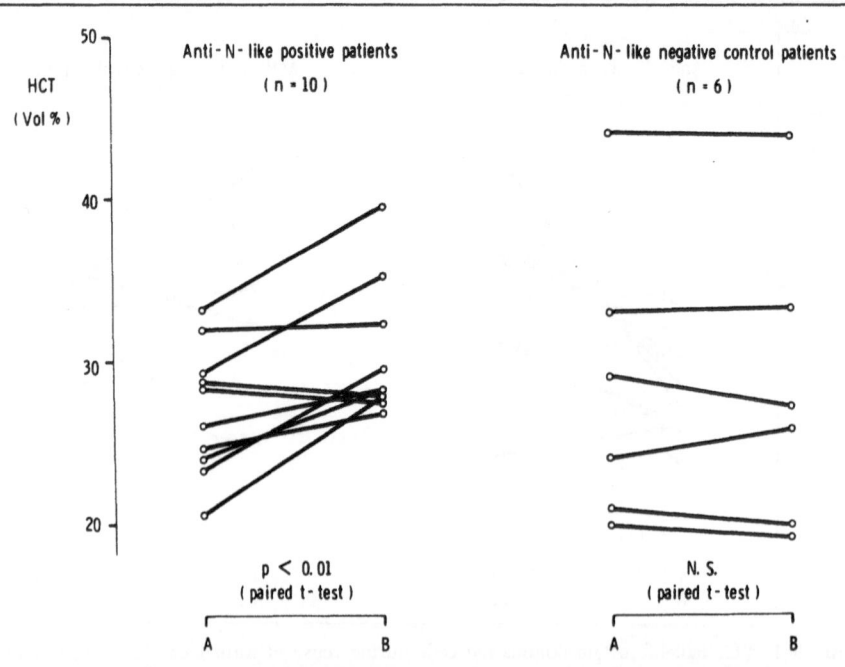

Figure 9-5. Hematocrit during reuse of formaldehyde-sterilized Kiil dialyzers (*A*) and subsequent single use of ethylene-oxide-sterilized disposable dialyzers (*B*). Reproduced, with permission, from *Trans Am Soc Artif Intern Organs* 24:709–712, 1978.

dialysis, when red cell half-life was measured, only minor changes occurred. At the end of the observation period of 6–14 months, however, titers were diminished by at least two doubling dilutions.

These data suggest that, in antibody-positive patients using formaldehyde-sterilized dialyzers, increased hemolysis does occur and that this hemolysis contributes to the anemia in these patients.

In agreement with Odgen et al. [18] and Lewis et al. [19], we have shown that our patients had been exposed to surprisingly high concentrations of formaldehyde at the start of dialysis. However, a significant direct hemolytic action of formaldehyde, as described by Orringer and Mattern [20], does not appear to have occurred. In antibody-negative patients, total avoidance of formaldehyde was accompanied by neither an increase of red cell life span nor hematocrit. Obviously, the role of formaldehyde in the pathogenesis of the observed hemolysis is more complex. We suggest the following concept (figure 9-7): In the first step, formaldehyde contact with red cells is a prerequisite for formation of the antibody [2, 3, 21–24], presumably by rendering the MN receptor immunogenic [3, 4]. As a consequence, in a second step, formation of the antibody will be induced in susceptible patients. In a third step, anti-N-like antibodies destroy erythrocytes bearing the formaldehyde-induced neoantigen.

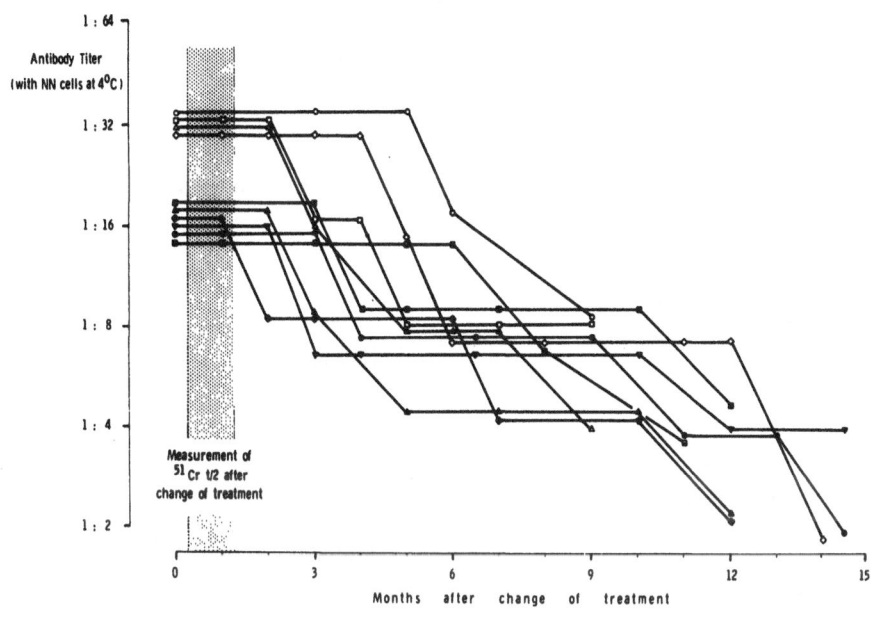

Figure 9-6. The effect of replacement of formaldehyde-sterilized Kiil dialyzers by ethylene-oxide-sterilized disposable dialyzers on anti-N-like antibody titers in hemodialysis patients (*n*=10). Reproduced, with permission, from *Trans Am Soc Artif Intern Organs* 24:709–712, 1978.

CRITICAL RESIDUAL FORMALDEHYDE CONCENTRATION

Further studies were performed to evaluate the critical residual formaldehyde concentration. As we had demonstrated, formaldehyde induces a dose-dependent alteration of the red cell membrane that makes the erythrocytes more susceptible to formation of anti-N-like antibodies. Figure 9-8 shows the results of more recent experiments where the red cells were preincubated with formaldehyde for 60 min at 37°C instead of 22°C as in earlier studies. This change of temperature was necessary to adjust the in vitro conditions to the situation at the start of dialysis. As can be seen, the strength of red cell agglutination by anti-N-like positive sera, expressed here in scores [25], is increased when the pretreatment formaldehyde concentration rises. The minimal formaldehyde concentration capable of inducing an effect was found to be 1.0 mg/dl. This suggests that reduction of hemolysis or even prevention of antibody formation can be achieved not only by total avoidance of formaldehyde as sterilant but also by reducing the formaldehyde concentration in the blood and dialysate compartments at the start of dialysis to values below 1.0 mg/dl.

Orringer and Mattern [20] found a decreased ATP content of erythrocytes exposed to a formaldehyde concentration of greater than 1.0 mg/dl, again suggesting this level as a possible critical value.

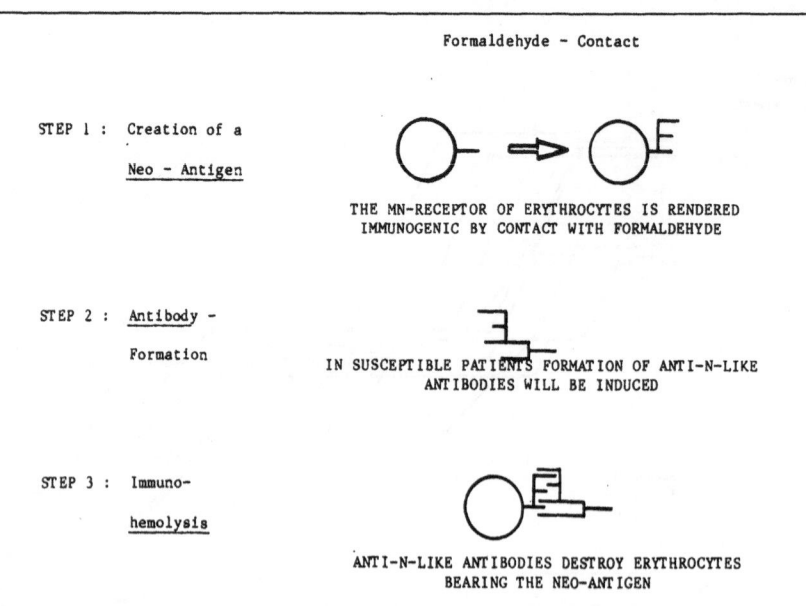

Figure 9-7. Suggested pathogenesis of formaldehyde-induced immunohemolysis due to anti-N-like antibodies.

AVOIDANCE OF ANTI-N-LIKE ANTIBODIES BY STERILANT REMOVAL

In 1981, Lewis et al. [26] confirmed that residual formaldehyde concentrations below 1 mg/dl do not induce the formation of anti-N-like antibodies. They determined irregular antibodies in two groups using formaldehyde-sterilized dialyzers. In one of the groups, due to a prolonged rinsing procedure of the dialyzers, this critical value was never exceeded. In this group, anti-N-like antibodies could not be detected.

We conclude that, by minimizing formaldehyde exposure, the occurrence of anti-N-like antibodies may be avoided in spite of the use of formaldehyde-sterilized dialyzers.

SUMMARY

The presence of anti-N-like antibodies in hemodialysis patients using formaldehyde-sterilized dialyzers is accompanied by increased hemolysis when the patient is exposed to critical residual concentrations of this sterilant. This increased hemolysis may contribute to the degree of anemia of these patients. When formaldehyde exposure of antibody-positive patients is totally avoided, red cell survival increases immediately. In contrast, antibody titers decline only gradually when formaldehyde is replaced as a dialyzer sterilant.

When formaldehyde is used, patients' exposure should be minimized by improving the rinsing technique and sensitivity of formaldehyde detection methods. These techniques and methods are readily available.

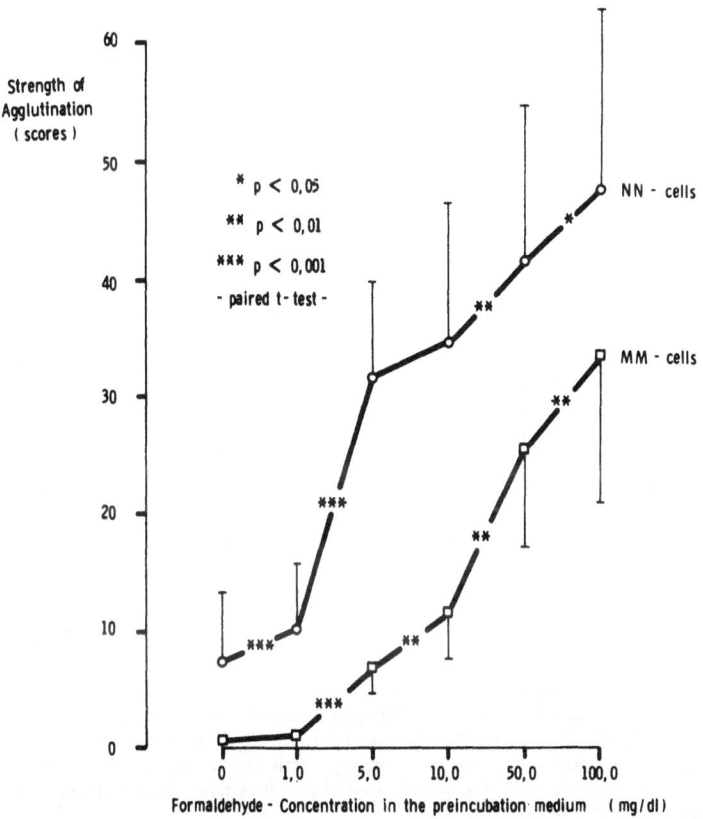

Figure 9-8. Formaldehyde pretreatment of erythrocytes (37°C for 1.0 h) and agglutinability by anti-N-like-positive sera ($n=6$). The effect of formaldehyde pretreatment concentration. Values shown are mean ± SD. Reproduced, with permission, from *Trans Am Soc Artif Intern Organs* 24:709–712, 1978.

Antibody formation and hemolysis can be prevented by reducing the formaldehyde concentration in the blood and dialysis compartment at the start of dialysis to values that are consistently below 1.0 mg/dl.

REFERENCES

1. Howell ED, Perkins HA: Anti-N-like antibodies in the sera of patients undergoing chronic hemodialysis. Vox Sang 23:291–299, 1972.
2. Harrison PB, Jansson K, Kronenberg H, Mahoney JG, Tiller D: Cold agglutinin formation in patients undergoing haemodialysis: a possible relationship to dialyser re-use. Aust NZ J Med 5:195–197, 1975.
3. Fassbinder W, Pilar J, Scheuermann E, Koch KM: Formaldehyde and the occurrence of anti-N-like cold agglutinins in RDT patients. Proc Eur Dial Transplant Assoc 13:333–338, 1976.
4. Fassbinder W, Seidl S, Koch KM: The role of formaldehyde in the formation of haemodialysis-associated anti-N-like antibodies. Vox Sang 35:41–48, 1978.
5. Pollard TL, Barnett BMS, Eschbach JW, Scribner BH: A technique for storage and multiple

re-use of the Kiil dialyzer and blood tubing. Trans Am Soc Artif Intern Org 13:24–28, 1967.

6. Nash T: The colorimetric estimation of formaldehyde by means of the Hantzsch reaction. Biochem J 55:416–421, 1953.
7. Winn LC, Eska PL, Grindon AJ: ABO discrepancy caused by an auto-anti-N. Transfusion 15:612–613, 1975.
8. Belzer FO, Kountz SL, Perkins HA: Red cell cold autoagglutinins as a cause of failure of renal allotransplantation. Transplantation 11:422–424, 1971.
9. Greenwalt TJ, Saski T, Steane EA: Second example of anti-N in a blood donor of group MN. Vox Sang 11:184–188, 1966.
10. Metaxas-Buhler M, Ikin EW, Romanski J: Anti-N in the serum of a healthy blood donor of group MN. Vox Sang 6:574–582, 1961.
11. Moores P, Botha MC, Brink S: Anti-N in the serum of a healthy type MN person: a further example. Am J Clin Pathol 54:90–93, 1970.
12. Perrault R: Naturally-occurring anti-M and anti-N with special case: IgG anti-N in a NN donor. Vox Sang 24:134–149, 1973.
13. Bowman HS, Marsh WL, Schumacher HR, Oyen R, Reihart J: Auto anti-N immunohemolytic anemia in infectious mononucleosis. Am J Clin Pathol 61:465–472, 1974.
14. Dube VE, House RF, Moulds J, Polesky HF: Hemolytic anemia caused by auto anti-N. Am J Clin Pathol 63:828–831, 1975.
15. Hinz CF, Boyer JT: Dysgammaglobulinemia in the adult manifested as autoimmune hemolytic anemia: serologic and immunochemical characterization of an antibody of unusual specificity. N Engl J Med 269:1329–1335, 1963.
16. Telischi M, Behzad O, Issitt PD, Pavone BG: Hemolytic disease of the newborn due to anti-N. Vox Sang 31:109–116, 1976.
17. Heimpel H: Hamatologie. In: Emrich D (ed) Nuklearmedizin Funktions-diagnostik. G Thieme, Stuttgart, 1971, pp 121–158.
18. Ogden DA, Myers LE, Eskelson CD, Ziegler EJ: Iatrogenic administration of formaldehyde to hemodialysis patients. Proc Dial Transplant Forum 5:141–145, 1973.
19. Lewis KJ, Ward MK, Kerr DNS: Residual formaldehyde in dialyzers: quantity, location, and the effect of different methods of rinsing. Artif Organs 5:269–277, 1981.
20. Orringer PE, Mattern WD: Formaldehyde-induced hemolysis during chronic hemodialysis. N Engl J Med 294:1416–1420, 1976.
21. Boettcher B, Nanra RS, Roberts TK, Mallan M, Watterson CA: Specificity and possible origin of anti-N antibodies developed by patients undergoing chronic hemodialysis. Vox Sang 31:408–415, 1976.
22. Crosson JT, Moulds J, Comty CM, Polesky HF: A clinical study of anti-N(DP) in the sera of patients in a large repetitive hemodialysis program. Kidney Int 10:463–470, 1976.
23. Kaehny WD, Miller GE, White WL: Relationship between dialyzer reuse and the presence of anti-N-like antibodies in chronic hemodialysis patients. Kidney Int 12:59–65, 1977.
24. Shaldon S, Chevallet M, Maraoui M, Mion C: Dialysis associated auto-antibodies. Proc Eur Dial Transplant Assoc 13:339–346, 1976.
25. Marsh WL: Scoring of hemagglutination reactions. Transfusion 12:352–353, 1972.
26. Lewis KJ, Dewar PJ, Ward MK, Kerr DNS: Formation of anti-N-like antibodies in dialysis patients: effect of different methods of dialyzer rinsing to remove formaldehyde. Clin Nephrol 15:39–43, 1981.

10. IMMUNE RESPONSE TO REUSE: ANAPHYLATOXINS AND IgE

LEE W. HENDERSON
DENNIS E. CHENOWETH

Two responses of the immune system have relevance for those interested in artificial kidney performance: first, those associated with complement activation and the release of anaphylatoxins and, second, those associated with immune complex formation and the type-I hypersensitivity reaction. Kaplow and Goffinet in 1972 [1] noted that profound leukopenia occurs within 30 min after initiating CUPROPHAN® hemodialysis. This phenomenon is now known to be the result of sequestration of polymorphonuclear leukocytes in the pulmonary microvasculative rather than on the dialysis membrane. It was noted early on that not all membranes cause this phenomenon [2, 3]. Increased polymorph adhesiveness is produced when certain types of dialyzer membranes activate the complement system with release of the anaphylatoxin C5a which binds to specific polymorph receptors. The type-I hypersensitivity reaction was brought into focus by the practice of membrane reuse and is considered as the most likely mechanism underlying one form of first-use syndrome.

What follows is a brief description of both the complement system and the IgE-mediated immune response, a comparative survey of the complement-activating properties of commonly used artificial kidney membranes, and an operating hypothesis as to the intimate blood–membrane events that trigger these reactions and how they may be influenced by reuse. Finally we will summarize presently available information about the clinical importance of

Deane, Wineman, and Bemis (eds.): GUIDE TO REPROCESSING OF HEMODIALYZERS.
© 1986. Martinus Nijhoff Publishing. All rights reserved.

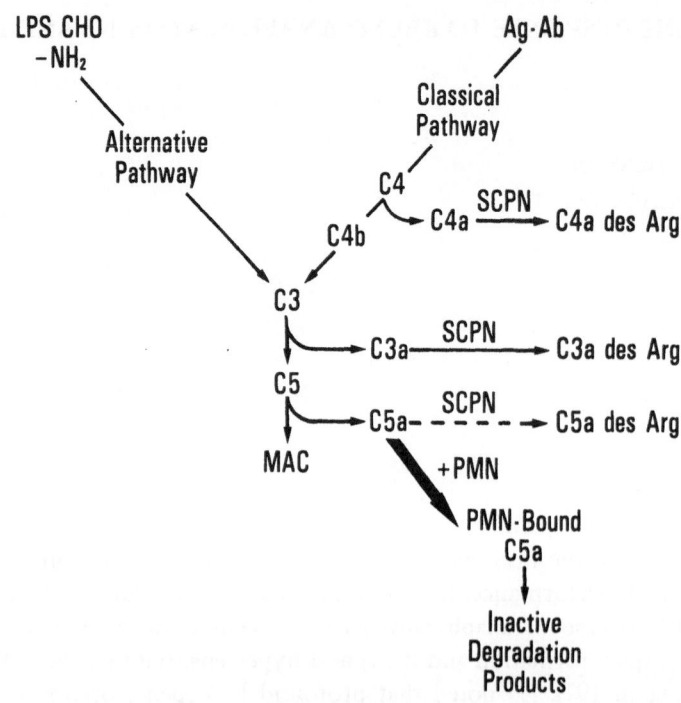

Figure 10-1. Diagram of the classic and alternative pathways of intravascular complement activation. Alternative pathway activation may occur as a result of exposure to a variety of substances including a carbohydrate (*CHO*) on cellulosic dialysis membrane. The anaphylatoxins *C4a* and *C5a* are converted to their *des Arg* form by a serum carboxypeptidase enzyme (*SCPN*). *C5a* is bound to the polymorphonuclear leukocyte (*PMN*). Downstream events include formation of the membrane attack complex (*MAC*).

complement activation and IgE-mediated responses in the end-stage renal disease patient.

THE COMPLEMENT SYSTEM

The human complement system consists of more than 20 plasma proteins normally found in blood as inactive molecules. When blood comes into contact with an appropriate stimulus, however, these inactive precursor molecules are enzymatically cleaved to yield bioactive proteins and polypeptides that contribute importantly to host defense mechanisms, i.e., they regulate the immune response, facilitate opsonization and phagocytosis, and function as critical mediators of the acute inflammatory response [4].

The activation of the complement cascade may proceed by two different mechanisms (figure 10-1). The first, termed the *classic pathway*, provides a specific means of immunosurveillance. Classic pathway activation is initiated when preformed antibodies bind to their target antigens. After this critical recognition step takes place, the classic pathway components C1, C4, and C2 assemble and undergo enzymatic cleavage. The second mechanism, termed the *alternative pathway*, provides a nonspecific means for the host to recognize "foreign" materials. According to current concepts, chemicals that act as nucleophiles may interact with a labile thiolester group on the active site of C3 to promote activation of this pathway. Regardless of the initiating stimulus, complement activation is characterized by C3 conversion to a low molecular weight polypeptide, C3a anaphylatoxin, that is released into the fluid phase. Subsequent cleavage of the next component in the complement scheme, C5, is deemed to be especially important because the low molecular weight glycopolypeptide C5a that is released from C5 is known to be an extremely potent mediator of granulocyte responses, including chemotaxis, adherence, aggregation, degranulation, and toxic oxygen radical production [5, 6, 7]. Normally, C5a would be expected to promote leukocyte accumulation and activation at local sites of inflammation and thus contribute to host defense. However, systemic or intravascular complement activation and C5a formation is thought to induce diffuse granulocyte activation that results in damage to multiple organ systems [4]. Precise quantitation of these anaphylatoxins is now possible using radioimmunoassay methodology.

TYPE-I HYPERSENSITIVITY

IgE-mediated immunologic events are usually classed as a type I or immediate hypersensitivity response. In general, individuals with no special predisposition to allergic reactions who sustain a type-I reaction are described as having an anaphylactic response whereas those who clearly show a predisposition to type-I reactions are described as having an atopic response. Type-I reactions do not occur on first exposure to an antigen, but rather on the second or subsequent exposures. The reason for this is that a first exposure of the individual to the antigen is required for there to be activation of helper T-lymphocytes that in turn stimulate specific B-lymphocytes to transform into antibody-producing plasma cells. The antibody is of the IgE variety and is specific for the antigens initiating the events. The antigen may be a protein or, in some instances, a smaller molecular weight chemical that acts as a hapten when attached to proteins. The IgE so formed binds to the surfaces of mast cells and basophils and, when the antigen is encountered for the second or subsequent time, immune complexes form on the surface of these cells. The presence of these complexes initiates a series of events within the cell that results in the release of powerful mediator substances that cause inflammation, e.g., histamine, bradykinin, slow-reacting substance of anaphylaxis, serotonin, and others. The clinical syndrome of anaphylaxis results, with the classic respiratory and dermatologic manifestations and capillary leak, cardiac rhythm change, shock and, at times, death.

The classic study tool to determine the presence of type-I hypersensitivity, i.e., the Prausuitz-Kustner reaction, has in large measure given way to the

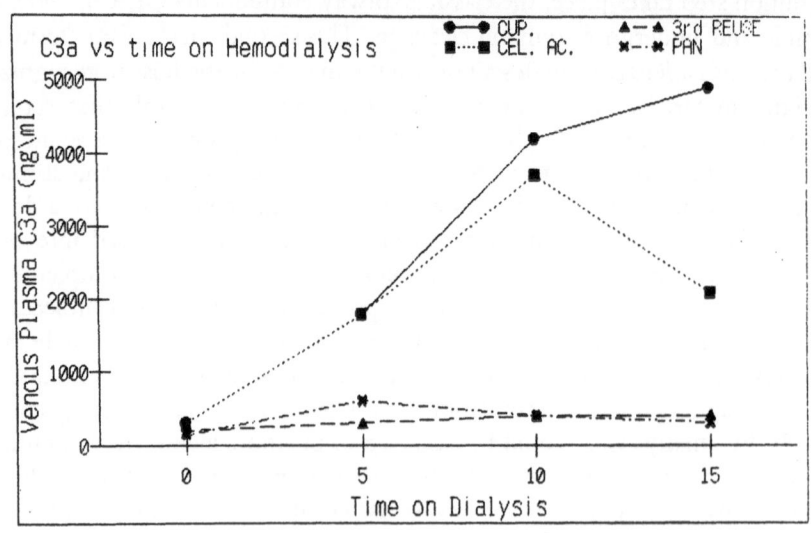

Figure 10-2. Venous plasma C3a levels plotted vs minutes on dialysis for new CUPROPHAN®
membrane (*solid circles*), CUPROPHAN® membrane that had been reused three times
(*closed triangles*), new cellulose acetate membrane (*closed squares*), and AN-69 PAN
membrane (*xs*). Reprinted by permission of the International Society for Artificial
Organs from Artificial Organs, 8:281-290, 1984.

radioallergosorbent test (RAST). This can provide a measure of the presence
of a specific IgE antibody to an offending antigen.

Some of the "downstream" mediators of the type-I hypersensitivity response are shared with those that result from the activation of the complement system. For example, release of the anaphylatoxin C5a can stimulate
mast cells to release histamine [8]. It is of interest that symptoms and signs
resulting from the activation of the complement system, while likely present,
are sufficiently subtle as to require a systematic investigation to differentiate
them from other dialysis–related events. Hence proof of their presence is only
now being sought, whereas the chemical events relating to the complement
system and its reaction to the dialysis membrane is fairly far advanced. This
is unlike the type-I hypersensitivity reaction, the clinical drama of which has
made its description clear in advance of delineation of the details of its plasma
and cell biochemistry.

COMPARATIVE SURVEY OF COMMONLY USED MEMBRANES

Figure 10-2 plots C3a concentration in the plasma of patients undergoing
hemodialysis vs time on dialysis for some commonly used hemodialysis [9]
membranes. It is apparent that cellulosic membrane is active in triggering
complement, whereas the noncellulosic AN-69 polyacrylonitrile membrane is
not. Of most importance is the observation that CUPROPHAN® membrane, the
most active of the widely used cellulosic membranes, is rendered inactive

after undergoing a saline rinse plus formaldehyde storage protocol as described in chapter 2. A recent report [10] indicates that a cellulose hydrate membrane is even more active than CUPROPHAN® in triggering complement. Other noncellulosic membranes, used primarily for hemofiltration, on first use are more comparable to PAN membrane. For example, the polysulfone membranes from Amicon (D-20, 30) and Fresenius (F-60), and the polyamide and polycarbonate membranes from Gambro, activate complement little if at all (L.W. Henderson and D.E. Chenoweth, unpublished observations).

AN HYPOTHESIS ON BLOOD–MEMBRANE INTERACTION

Description of the thiolester bond present at the active site on the C3 molecule and the comparative information on the different membranes noted above have led us to postulate that it is the hydroxyl group present on the cellulosic membrane that reacts with this bond, splitting it and initiating the downstream events of the complement cascade. The number of these hydroxyl groups on the membrane would then be an important determinant of the degree to which a membrane activates the system. From this hypothesis it is apparent that acetylation of these hydroxyl groups to form cellulose acetate would reduce the number of sites available for activation and would explain the lower curve noted in Figure 10-2 for this membrane. The PAN membrane with its nitrile rather than hydroxyl groups does not attack the thiolester bond. The amount of membrane surface area, how it is configured (number and length of parallel paths), as well as the tempo at which blood flow rate is increased on initiating treatment should all influence the degree to which an artificial kidney membrane will activate complement. At present none of these factors has received formal evaluation either clinically or in vitro.

THE IMPACT OF DIALYZER REUSE

Figure 10-3 plots the degree of in vivo C3a activation with time in new and serially reused 1.0-m² CUPROPHAN® dialyzers [11]. Figure 10-4 shows the corresponding data for the reduction in white blood cell counts [12]. As with first use of the membrane, there is an excellent correlation between C3a concentration in the plasma returning to the patient and the degree of leukopenia [12].

It should be noted that C3a measured in the returning blood is a better measure of the degree to which the membrane has activated complement than is the level of C5a, as the latter is swiftly bound to the polymorphs and monocytes and is unavailable for assay. It is noteworthy that there is little or no change in complement activation between the second and fifth reuse as contrasted with the large change from new to first reuse and of fifth reuse to new membrane.

We would explain the reduction in complement activation with reuse by postulating the binding of C3b- or C3b-derived fragments such as C3d to the

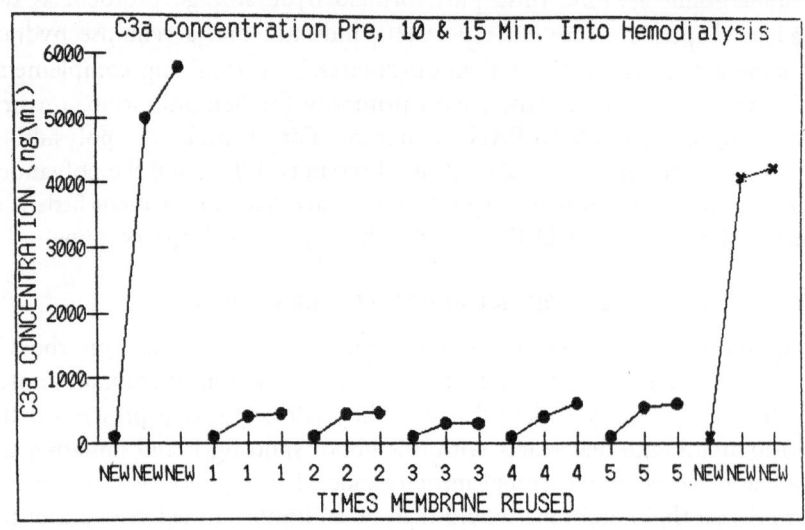

Figure 10-3. Serum concentrations of C3a are plotted prior to dialysis and at the 10- and 15-min mark for a new membrane, in subsequent reuse on five occasions (*closed circles*) and reintroduction of a new membrane (*x*s). The values given are averaged for the 11 subjects studied.

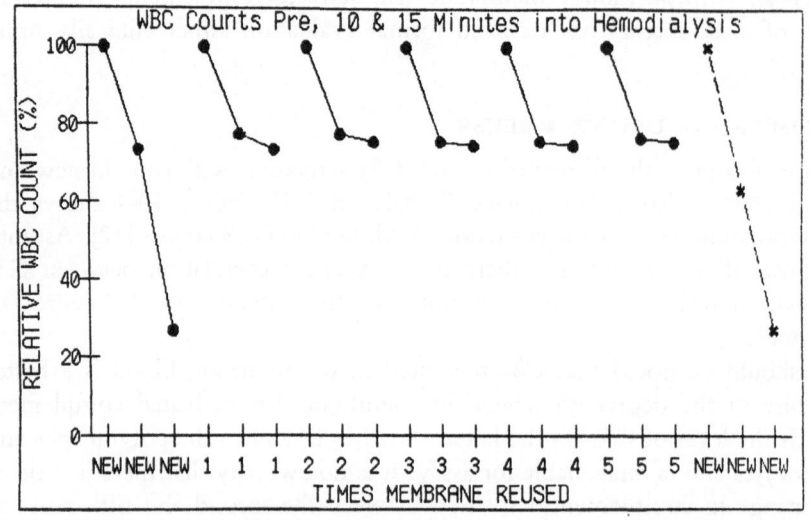

Figure 10-4. Relative white blood cell counts are plotted predialysis as well as at the 10- and 15-min mark for the 11 subjects studied in figure 10-3.

active sites on the membrane rather than the nonspecific binding of other plasma proteins such as albumin. This conclusion stems from our studies in which a reused dialyzer was perfused with a phosphate-buffered saline solution containing radiolabeled rabbit antihuman C3b antibodies. This dialyzer showed an uptake of antibody (73%) that was entirely comparable (68%) to the positive control (a sepharose 4B column to which C3b antigen had been attached) [11, 12]. Two negative controls were run. The first was a new CUPROPHAN® dialyzer prepared as if for clinical use and identical to those used for the first part of the experiment. The second was an unused dialyzer that was formalin fixed using the protocol employed for the reused membrane. Both showed comparable but markedly less uptake of the antibody (23%). This lack of uptake in the formalin-treated control coupled with the clinical observation of a significant fall in white blood cell count and elevation in venous line C3a concentration with formaldehyde-treated new membrane points strongly away from formaldehyde as playing a role in the reduced level of complement activation with reused membrane. Recent work by Stroncek et al. [13] supports this position.

A recent report identifies that when a CUPROPHAN® dialyzer is cleaned with sodium hypochlorite for reuse, full complement activating potential is restored [14]. This observation would be compatible with a more thorough cleaning if not etching of the membrane by this agent with removal of the C3b- and C3b-derived proteins from the active sites on the membrane surface.

So far there are no studies reported on the effects of alternate sterilants (as described in chapter 2) on either restoring the complement-activating properties of the membrane or activating complement by their trace presence in the system.

CLINICAL CORRELATES OF IMMUNOLOGICALLY MEDIATED REPONSE TO ARTIFICIAL KIDNEY MEMBRANES

With the upswing in membrane reuse, clinicians involved in this practice became aware of a first-use syndrome [15] that because of its clinical severity has captured national attention and been the subject of an epidemiologic study by the FDA [16]. This first-use syndrome, because of its clinical similarity to allergy/anaphylaxis, is considered likely to be a type-I hypersensitivity reaction, i.e., wheal and erythemia, bronchospasm, rhinorrhea, tearing, and at times shock and death, as well as response to treatment with antihistamines, steroids, and norepinephrine. For clarity, this definition will be referred to as first-use syndrome 1 (FUS-1). A second definition (FUS-2), which workers such as Hakim et al. [17], Robson et al. [118], and others have introduced into the literature, describes an increase in intratreatment morbidity that is not clearly an allergic manifestation nor limited to the first hour of dialysis. It encompasses all of the symptoms and signs associated with routine dialysis. Death is quite unusual with FUS-2.

Villarroel [16] has tabulated the incidence of FUS-1, which he subgrades into mild, moderate, and severe (death), and identifies a low overall frequency, i.e., 3−4 episodes/100,000 hollow-fiber dialyzers sold. This, like most adverse reactions, is probably underreported, and hence the incidence given may be considered a minimum. Most FUS-1 incidents are associated with the use of CUPROPHAN® hollow-fiber membranes. Sheet CUPROPHAN® membrane and CUPROPHAN® tubes (coil dialyzer) show a lower incidence as do noncellulosic (PAN, polysulfone, polyamide) membranes. At present, the underlying etiology in terms of an antigen for FUS-1 remains obscure. Evidence bearing on its etiology has centered mostly heavily on an IgE-mediated reaction to some constituent of the dialyzer. Ethylene oxide residual and/or limulus amoebocyte lysate (LAL) reactive, nonpyrogenic material (thought to be the result of residual products of the linters used in the preparation of the CUPROPHAN®) lead the list of suspected antigens [19−21]. Why membrane in sheet or tube form is different in this respect from that in hollow-fiber format is not as yet clear. Radioallergosorbent testing (RAST) has been reported to be positive against ethylene oxide in 12% of dialysis patients, but it failed to correlate closely with that of FUS-1. A high incidence is reported by Sherlock and Olmer (39%), but again there was no correlation with clinical symptoms [22]. Eosinophilia, also noted to be common in dialysis patients, has also not been shown to correlate either with a positive RAST test or with FUS-1 occurrence [22]. The low incidence of FUS-1 hampers an orderly and prospective study of patients exhibiting this syndrome. It is the common clinical wisdom that patients switched from treatment with other membranes and/or membrane formats constitute the major population at risk for FUS-1. It is noteworthy that residual ethylene oxide and/or LAL reactive material should be eliminated with the preuse rinsing procedures recommended by the manufacturer. One line of speculation notes that hollow-fiber CUPROPHAN® requires potting compound at either end such as polyurethane whereas this is not true for coils and a commonly used sheet membrane format (Gambro Lundia). One may then further speculate that some constituent of the potting compound including absorbed ethylene oxide may underlie the expression of FUS-1. An alternative explanation that is less readily reconciled with the clinical observations is to postulate an exaggerated response (excessive generation or impaired degradation) of the complement system or to its breakdown products C3a and C5a known to have anaphylatoxic properties that is individual specific. Why comparable membrane area in different formats would result in a different incidence is not addressed by this hypothesis. More information is needed before we can explain in detail the pathophysiologic events of FUS-1. By definition, FUS-1 does not occur with reused membrane.

Information on the pathophysiology of FUS-2 links it more closely with complement-related events, but again these data are inferential rather than direct. In a study of patients undergoing cardiopulmonary bypass, the statistical correlation between such morbid events as the occurrence of renal failure and death showed a strong positive correlation with the level of plasma C3a at the conclusion of the procedure. Additionally, Hakim et al. [17] showed that in a group of ESRD patients, selected because they had high incidence of intratreatment morbid events, both a higher (approximately 30%) and earlier peak of plasma C3a concentration occurred during dialysis than in their less symptomatic counterparts. Studies reported in abstract support the FUS-2 definition by demonstrating a higher incidence of intratreatment morbid events in end-stage renal disease patients exposed to new dialysis membranes as compared with those using a saline rinse formalin storage protocol [18]. This information, taken in light of the diminished activation of complement in the saline/formalin reused membrane, again shows a correlation but not necessarily an etiologic relationship between these phenomena. The observations that peak anaphylatoxin release occurs in less than 20 min in most patients and that symptomatic hypotension more commonly peaks in incidence in the third and fourth hours of treatment are difficult to reconcile. The hypothesis that complement activation, in particular the release of C5a and its interaction with the monocyte, may beget interleukin-1 (IL-1) has been put forward [23]. This hypothesis further suggests that IL-1 via the arachidonic acid pathway mediates not only an acute phase response but underlies the vascular instability associated with intratreatment morbidity. Studies in sheep and swine identify profound changes in cardiovascular state and in particular correlate profound increase in pulmonary artery pressure with the presence of C5a in the circulation and its presumed triggering of "downstream" events in the complement cascade that release the potent vasoconstrictor thromboxane A2 [24]. There is conflicting information in man with Walker et al. [25] reporting an increase in pulmonary artery pressure analogous to that seen in the animal models while Bergstrom et al. [26] fail to identify this change in nonuremic study subjects on sham (no dialysate circulating) CUPROPHAN® dialysis. Again, more information is necessary to permit full understanding of these interesting correlations.

Lastly, Yudis et al. have reported a patient who exhibits an adverse response to reused membranes [27]. Concern about formaldehyde infusions and, in addition, the denaturing of protein absorbed to the membrane in such a manner as to make it antigenic either via a hapten mechanism or simply by profound conformational changes has long been with us. This first reporting of a second-use syndrome bears our attention as the practice of reuse becomes increasingly more common [28].

CONCLUSIONS

At present then, we note that the practice of dialyzer reuse is strongly increasing in the United States, that for a saline rinse/formaldehyde storage protocol with CUPROPHAN® membrane, complement activation is less than with unused membrane and, by definition, that FUS-1 does not occur with reuse. We do not have a clear etiologic link between clinical morbidity (either FUS-1 or FUS-2) and complement activation either during treatment or chronically although recent studies suggest such a link. We also do not understand the underlying pathophysiology of FUS-1. Further studies will be necessary in order to determine the impact of membrane reuse on these immunologic events as well as on the organism as a whole over time.

REFERENCES

1. Kaplow LS, Goffinet JA: Profound neutropenia during the early phase of hemodialysis. JAMA 203:1135–1137, 1968.
2. Henderson LW, Miller ME, Hamilton RW, Norman ME: Dialysis leukopenia polymorph random mobility and the control of peripheral white blood cell levels: a preliminary observation. J Lab Clin Med 85:191–197, 1975.
3. Aljama P, Bird PAE, Ward MK, Feest TG, Walker W, Tanboga H, Sussman M, Kerr DNS: Hemodialysis induced leukopenia and activation of complement: effects of different membranes. Proc Eur Dial Transplant Assoc 15:144–151, 1978.
4. Atkinson JP, Frank MM: In: Parker CW (ed) Clinical immunology. CW Parker (editor) WB Saunders, Philadelphia, 1980, pp 219–271.
5. Chenoweth DE, Hugli TE: Demonstration of specific C5a receptor on intact human polymorphonuclear leukocytes. Proc Natl Acad Sci USA:3943–3947, 1978.
6. Chenoweth DE, Hugli TE: Human C5a and C5a analogs as probes of the neutrophil C5a receptor. Mol Immunol 17:151–161, 1980.
7. Jacob HS: Complement-mediated leukoembolization: a mechanism of tissue damage during extracorporeal perfusions, myocardial infarction and in shock—a review. Q J Med 52:289–296, 1983.
8. Johnson AR, Hugli TE, Muller-Eberhard HJ: Release of histamine from rat mast cells by the complement peptides C3a and C5a. Immunology 28:1067–1071, 1975.
9. Chenoweth DE: Complement activation during hemodialysis: clinical observations, proposed mechanisms and theoretical implications. Artif Organs 8:281–290, 1984.
10. Amadori A, Candi P, Sasdelli M, Massai G, Favilla S, Passaleva A, Ricci M: Hemodialysis leukopenia and complement function with different dialyzers. Kidney Int 24:775–781, 1983.
11. Chenoweth DE, Cheung AK, Ward DM, Henderson LW: Anaphylatoxin formation during hemodialysis: comparison of new and reused dialyzers. Kidney Int 24:770–774, 1983.
12. Chenoweth DE, Cheung AK, Henderson LW: Anaphylatoxin formation during hemodialysis: effects of different dialyzer membranes. Kidney Int 24:764–769, 1983.
13. Stroncek DF, Kesheviah P, Craddock PR, Hammerschmidt DE: Effect of dialyzer reuse on complement activation and neutropenia in hemodialysis. J Lab Clin Med 104:304–311, 1984.
14. Jayashankar JE, Karfonta S, Venkatachalam K, Deegan MJ, Duschene M, Zasuwa G, Levin NW: Effect of method of dialyzer reprocessing on complement activation: leukopenia and symptoms during hemodialysis—randomized controlled study [abstr]. Am Soc Artif Intern Organs 31st Annu Meet, 1985, p 57.
15. Ogden DA: New-dialyzer syndrome [letter]. N Engl J Med 302:1262, 1980.
16. Villarroel F: Incidence of hypersensitivity in hemodialysis. Artif Organs 8:278–280, 1984.
17. Hakim RM, Breillatt J, Lazarus JM, Port FK: Complement activation and hypersensitivity reactions to dialysis membranes. N Engl J Med 311:878–882, 1984.
18. Robson M, Pollak VE, Kant KS, Charoenpanich R, Cathey M: There is a syndrome associated with the use of new dialyzers [abstr]. Am Soc Nephrol 17th Annu Meet, 1984, p 72.
19. Dolovich J, Marshall CP, Smith EKM, Shimizu A, Pearson FC, Sugona MA, Lee W: Allergy to ethylene oxide in chronic hemodialysis patients. Artif Organs 8:334–337, 1984.
20. Butcher BT, Reed MA, O'Neill CE, Leech S, Pearson FC: Immunologic studies of hollow-fiber dialyzer extracts. Artif Organs 8:318–328, 1984.
21. Henne W, Schulze H, Pelger M, Tretzel J, Von Sengbusch G: Hollow-fiber dialyzers and their pyrogenicity testing by limulus amebocyte lysate. Artif Organs 8:299–305, 1984.

22. Sherlock J, Olmer J: Immediate hypersensitivity to dialyzer contents [abstr]. Am Soc Nephrol 17th Annu Meet, 1984, p 742.
23. Henderson LW, Koch KM, Dinarello CA, Shaldon S: Hemodialysis hypotension: the interleukin hypothesis. J Blood Purification 1:3–8, 1984.
24. Cheung AK, Baranowski RL: The role of thromboxane in pulmonary hypertension induced by cuprophan-activated plasma [abstr]. Am Soc Nephrol 17th Annu Meet, 1984, p 60.
25. Walker JF, Lindsay RM, Driedger AA, Sibbald WJ, Linton AL: Hemodialysis commonly causes transient pulmonary hypertension [abstr]. Kidney Int 25:195, 1984.
26. Bergstrom J, Danielsson A, Freyschuss U: Dialysis ultrafiltration and sham-dialysis in normal subjects [abstr]. Am Soc Nephrol 17th Annu Meet, 1984, p 59.
27. Yudis M, Sirota RA, Stein HD: Dialyzer hypersensitivity reaction associated with reuse [abstr]. Am Soc Artif Intern Organs 31st Annu Meet, 1985, p 59.
28. Bland L, Alter M, Favero M, Carson L, Cusick L: Hemodialyzer reuse: practices in the United States and implications for infection control [abstr]. Am Soc Artif Intern Organs 31st Annu Meet, 1985, p 40.

11. AUTOMATED REPROCESSING

ROBERT J. WINEMAN

The year 1985 is recognized as the 25th anniversary of the application of hemodialysis on a chronic basis to outpatients. In the first few years of outpatient hemodialysis, manual processes for the reuse of disposable coil and flat-plate Kiil dialyzers originated [1, 2]. By the mid-1970s, a number of reports were available on the development of automated devices to perform rinsing and resterilization of hemodialyzers [3, 4]. Certain early devices were modifications of single-station dialysate delivery systems that provided the capability for rinsing and sterilizing the hemodialyzer at the same time as the dialysate delivery machine was being sterilized. Such developments were primarily directed to the home dialysis patient.

On the other hand, other early devices were free-standing automated machines for conducting the steps for dialyzer reprocessing similar to a manual procedure. Examples are the Ma-De 100 [3] and the dialyzer cleaning machine developed by Hardy and associates [5]. In the late 1970s and early 1980s, primarily in the United States, a number of such dedicated devices were developed. The development of the manual reprocessing steps of rinsing, cleaning, testing, and disinfection (see chapter 2) helped to lay the ground work for development of automated devices to perform these functions [6]. By the early 1980s, six such dedicated devices were on the market in the United States.

In a 1984 survey of the status of hemodialyzer reuse in the United States conducted by the Renal Physicians Association (see chapter 1), some form of automated reprocessing was utilized by 39.5% of all facilities that reprocessed hemodialyzers; 58% of such facilities utilized manual procedures exclusively, while 2.5% did not specify. According to this survey the mean number of uses of hemodialyzers for facilities using manual procedures was 8.2 ± 3.3 compared with facilities that used automated devices with documentation whose average number of uses was 9.1 ± 3.8. The group of facilities that are utilizing more simple reprocessing devices (without automated documentation) reported a mean number of reuses of 6.9 ± 2.2 [7].

EARLY APPLICATIONS OF AUTOMATED DEVICES

In 1974, Alberttazzi and coworkers [8] reported the development of a four-station automated dialyzer reprocessing machine. This device alternately applied pressurized, deionized water to the blood compartment followed by a vacuum of 15 mm mercury pressure in rapid sequence, such that 20−30 cycles could be completed in each 4- to 6-min cleaning process. Formaldehyde in 0.5% concentration was used as the disinfectant. While the device was said to be equally applicable to the flat plate, coil, or hollow fiber, data are presented only on hollow-fiber artificial kidneys, wherein fiber bundle volume losses of approximately 20% were experienced in 11 uses, with a corresponding loss of clearance of small molecules.

A prototype of a single-station device, called the Ma-De 100, which could be used to reprocess coil, flat-plate, or hollow-fiber dialyzers and their blood lines, was described by De Palma and coworkers [3]. The machine consisted of a disposable cartridge containing tubing and pump segments that could be fitted into a valve assembly and timing device that constituted the main part of the machine. The process utilized rinsing, cleaning, and disinfecting cycles that could be varied by the user. The disinfectant was formaldehyde while peroxide was utilized as a cleaning agent in overall suggested cycle times of 30−50 min. Qualitative results are reported to be satisfactory.

The dialyzer rinsing machine developed by Ahmad and Goldsmith in the United Kingdom was made commerically available by the Dylade Company [4]. This device offered adjustable cycles for rinsing the dialyzer and blood lines with either tapwater, 1% sodium hypochlorite, or 3% formalin. Initial applications were for reuse of Kiil dialyzers or Gambro disposable flat-plate dialyzers.

Another automated cycling device for reprocessing of hemodialyzers was developed in Canada and reported in 1976 by Hardy and coworkers [5]. This device utilized 3% hydrogen peroxide as the cleaning agent and formaldehyde as a disinfectant. Cycle times were 17−20 min with hollow-fiber and/or parallel-plate hemodialyzers. When used over a period of 18 months, an average of 3.05 uses was obtained with machine processed dialyzers compared with 2.7 uses with a manual technique. Overall costs were lower for the automated procedure than with the manual due primarily to the cost of technician time. Marketing rights for the machine were assigned to Drake-

Willock Systems. Higgins and coworkers [9] reported a clinical study of six patients using this device for reprocessing of Gambro-Lundia 13.5-micron flat-plate dialyzers. No significant differences were found in the in vivo small molecule clearances between the first use versus the third or fifth use. No significant reduction in in vitro BSP clearances or reduction in ultrafiltration rates occurred.

An automated reuse station was also developed by Vandenbroucke and coworkers of Belgium for reprocessing flat-plate hemodialyzers [10]. The Gambro Major and RP-6 hemodialyzers were studied. In the case of the RP-6, which has a polyacrylonitrile membrane (AN-69), it was possible to use sodium hypochlorite as both the cleaning agent and sterilant. The Gambro Major was cleaned with sodium hypochlorite solution and then rinsed and sterilized with 4% formaldehyde. Over ten uses could be achieved with no difference in efficiency for the RP-6 dialyzer, but the Gambro Major showed reduced clearances of small molecules of approximately 15%−20% in seven uses. Vandenbroucke and coworkers found that the efficiency of reuse was highly dependent on the delay between completion of dialysis and rinsing. When delay exceeded 30 min, small molecule clearances fell by 20% after seven uses, compared with less than 10% when the delay was below 10 min.

The Dylade model DS reuse system is a single-station dialysate delivery system that was modified to rinse and disinfect hemodialyzers following use. This device was marketed by the Milton Roy Company. It also functioned to prepare the hemodialyzer for the next clinical use following storage by automatically providing a treated water rinse of the dialysate compartment to aid in formaldehyde removal. Fitzcharles and coworkers conducted an evaluation of the Dylade DS using a mix of hemodialyzer types. It was found that no dialyzer lost more than 6% creatinine clearance in three or six uses. No significant impairment of performance occurred in ultrafiltration capability, nor was there any incidence of blood leaks or ruptured membranes [11].

An automated device (ABG 74, manufactured by ABG-Semca of Paris) was utilized by Man and associates to reuse hemodialyzers without formaldehyde [12, 13]. The dialyzers reused were RP-6 dialyzers, which had polyacrylonitrile (AN-69) membranes. Following dialysis, the hemodialyzers were both cleaned and sterilized with 0.67% sodium hypochlorite solution, which was pumped through the dialyzer at a flow rate of 500 ml/min. In a 45-patient clinical study comparing reuse (35 patients) with no reuse (ten patients), no anti-N-like antibodies were detected in either group. The conclusion is drawn that reuse per se does not cause such antibody formation. A further feature of the ABG 74 is that it may be used to rinse formaldehyde from a stored dialyzer prior to its use for the next dialysis. Lewis and coworkers caution that, as programmed in 1980, the rinse out was quite inadequate [14].

A prototype dialyzer reprocessing machine, developed and tested by Gentles and coworkers [15], had as its primary feature a built-in system for evaluation of membrane compliance, so that incipient failure of the membrane would be apparent to the operator. Otherwise, the device utilized peroxide for cleaning, various rinse cycles, and formaldehyde sterilization. Results of a clinical evaluation gave an average number of uses of dialyzers of 3.4, with less than 10% reduction in small molecule (in vivo) and larger solute (in vitro) clearances [16].

EFFECTS OF AUTOMATED PROCESSING ON BIOCOMPATIBILITY OF HEMO-DIALYZERS

To avoid some of the disadvantages of formaldehyde, Bauer and coworkers [17] conducted an evaluation of peracetic acid as both a cleaning agent and sterilant for reprocessing hemodialyzers. For cleaning a solution of 0.07% peracetic acid was utilized, while for disinfection the concentration was 0.025%. The investigators used a Renatron automated reuse machine (Renal Systems) for this study. In vitro and in vivo clearances were not significantly different for small molecules for new and reprocessed hemodialyzers. The dialyzers studied were Fresenius/Dylade Hemoflow D2 hollow fiber dialyzers with CUPROPHAN® membranes. In this somewhat limited study, observations were that no leukopenia occurred early in dialysis after storage of the hemodialyzer with peracetic acid as both sterilant and, earlier, as a cleaning agent. This behavior is in contrast to observations of others [17, 18] when sodium hypochlorite was employed as a cleaning agent.

In an investigation of a number of factors concerning function and biocompatibility of reused hemodialyzers, Hoenich and associates employed both manual and automated reuse procedures [18]. Flat-plate hemodialyzers were reprocessed by the commercially available automated system ABG-Semca type 704S (ABG Semca, S.A.) in which the hemodialyzer blood compartment is cleaned by rinsing with 0.5% sodium hypochlorite solution in a pulsed flow mode, followed by a rinse with 2% formaldehyde and finally a filling phase in which both compartments are filled with 2% formaldehyde. The investigators observed that use of sodium hypochlorite for cleaning the membrane caused the typical hemodialysis leukopenia to occur with the reprocessed hemodialyzer in essentially the same manner as with a new hemodialyzer. In contrast, rinsing or cleaning with reverse osmosis water provided dialyzers that demonstrated very little depression in white count early in dialysis. When studied through six uses, no marked deterioration in clearance properties or other functional characteristics of the dialyzers occurred when dialyzers were reprocessed either manually or by the automated procedures.

In another study of automated compared with manual reprocessing of hemodialyzers, Gagnon and Kaye observed that the concentration of the cleaning agent was the critical factor determining whether the hemodialyzer would cause typical hemodialysis leukopenia after reprocessing. In this study the automated reprocessing device was a Lixivitron II, in which hemodialyzers are subjected to a 5-s bleach cycle using sodium hypochlorite at 4.3% concentration. In contrast, the manual procedure utilized 1.0% sodium hypochlorite, which did not cause marked changes in the circulating neutrophil count. This observation was confirmed by other experiments using an entirely manual reprocessing procedure to compare 1% hypochlorite versus 4.2% hypochlorite. The results were similar; namely, the 1% hypochlorite was associated with very little change in neutrophil count in subsequent use of the reprocessed dialyzer, while 4.3% hypochlorite caused typical hemodialysis neutropenia [19]. (See also chapters 6, 9, and 10.)

DEVICES AVAILABLE IN THE UNITED STATES FOR AUTOMATED REPROCESSING

The information provided in this section was made available with the cooperation of the device manufacturers. Because of the limitations of space and the time-sensitive nature of machine features and prices, readers are advised to contact manufacturers directly for the most current data on devices of interest.

Please refer to table 11-1 in which various features of the devices are tabulated. The comments concerning each device are supplementary to the table and do not repeat the tabulated data.

Single-station devices

The Echo reprocessing device is made by Mesa Medical, Inc. of Littleton, Colorado. With the Center Echo machine, use of a cleaning agent such as sodium hypochlorite or hydrogen peroxide is optional. The Echo has also been approved for several other sterilants such as gluteraldehyde (CIDEX®, SPOROCIDIN®), WAREXIN®, in addition to 2% and 4% formaldehyde. The cycle may be customized but typically a cleaning process consists of a reverse ultrafiltration step, followed by a rinse and an optional peroxide cleaning step, with a further rinse prior to testing. Tests consist of a pressure leak test, and a cell volume measurement, which must be read visually by the operator. For a positive check for presence of sterilant, a sample is made available for external testing. Mesa Medical markets two other versions of reprocessing devices. The company should be consulted for details.

The Renatron, manufactured by Renal Systems of Minneapolis, Minnesota, is a single-station dialyzer reprocessing device that can employ either formaldehyde as a sterilant/disinfectant or RENALIN® as the cleaning agent/sterilant. RENALIN® is a formulation of peracetic acid. A simplified model for use by the home patient is also marketed by Renal Systems. The process consists of a series of rinses prior to a cleaning step utilizing RENALIN® followed by additional rinses and a test phase. Any dialyzer passing the tests (cell volume and leak) is automatically filled with the sterilant/disinfectant. In Bauer's experience with the Renatron [17] cited earlier, hemodialyzers were reused up

Table 11-1. Features of automated reprocesing devices

Device/features	Mesa Center Echo	Renatron with RENALIN®	Seratronics DRS 4	Texas Medical ADR-22	Harco Med Lixivitron II	Compudial KP-1
Installation						
Size WxHxD (cm)	38×46×56	37×41×31	76×122×71	56×174×66	118×171×98	123×170×73
Stations	1	1	4	4	4[a]	4–12
Treated water						
Reg l-min	1.5	1.75AV	1.5	1.5	3.9	1.0
Pressure (min) psi	40	20	30	20	20	20
Ventilation	–	"not required"	+	–	–	+
Sink rinse	Optional	–	+	–	+	+
Drain (l/min)	2	6	2	2	4	3.8
Process						
Cleaning agent	Optional	RENALIN®	NaOCl	H O (0.5%)	NaOCl	NaOCl
Cycle time (min)	8–20	7.5	28/4	35/4	20/4	20/4
Sterilant/disinfectant	2% HCHO or other See text	RENALIN®	1.5%–4% HCHO	4% HCHO or gluteraldehyde	2.7%–4% HCHO	2.6%–4% HCHO
Reverse UF	+	+	+	+	+	+
Rinse	+	+	+	+	+	+
Clean	+	+	+	+	+	+
Test	+	+	+	+	+	+
Disinfect	+	+	+	+	+	+
Tests						
Pressure leak	+	+	+	+	+	+
Cell volume	+ (Visually read)	+	+	+	+	+ (Optional)

KUF	–	–	+	+	+	+
Hemoglobin	–	–	+	–	–	+
Dialyzer identification	–	–	Bar code	Bar code	Bar code	Key
Positive test for disinfection	See text	–	+	+	–	+
Automated documentation	–	–	+	+	+	+
Statistics	–	–	+	+	+	+
Machine sanitizing		RENALIN®				
Cleaning Cycle	+	RENALIN®	+	+	+	+
Sterilization	(See text)	(See text)	+	+	+	+ 2.6%–4% HCHO
Maintenance						
Factory	+ (See text)	+	–	+	–	+
Regional	+	–	+	–	+	–
Ann. contract	–	+	+	?	+	+
Ann. contract cost $US	470–750	NA	2000	?	6600	4000
Maintenance seminar	+	+	+	+	+	+
Diagnostics via modem	–	–	+	–	–	+
Notes of other features		Home model	Test limits to phys. prescrip.			
Can be customized	+	+		+	?	+
Cleared for other sterilants	+	Version sold for HCHO	CIDEX®	Gluteraldehyde	?	CIDEX®
List price ($1000 US)	4.7–5.7	8.5	40	39.5	64	30.40
List price/station ($1000 US)	4.7–5.7	8.5	10	9.5	16	3.3–7.5

aHarco also markets a two-station unit.

to six times with no adverse intradialytic effects like fever, chills, headache, or bacteremia.

The single-station reprocessing devices discussed above, the Echo and Renatron, were originally directed toward both in-center and home patients applications. Now each company has special units for the home patients. Utilizing a different approach, Colorado Medical Corporation has developed a single patient dialyzer reuse device, the HR3000, which operates in conjunction with a single patient dialysate delivery system to reprocess dialyzers and blood tubing sets. The HR3000 conducts a cleaning cycle utilizing 0.25% sodium hypochlorite, a rinse cycle followed by disinfection cycle. The machine also functions to prepare the dialyzer for subsequent use by rinsing out the formaldehyde disinfectant. A pass–fail clearance test is conducted based on the clearance of sodium chloride being between ± 20% of the nominal value for the dialyzer being used. In a detailed clinical evaluation of the device, Ogden and Friedl found that urea and creatinine clearances were maintained in excess of 90% of the values of the new hemodialyzers, while B12 clearances and KUF increased significantly over 18 uses [20].

Multistation devices

The Seratronics DRS-4 is a multistation dialyzer reprocessing machine manufactured by Seratronics of Concord, California. This machine employs bleach as a cleaning agent and formaldehyde as a sterilant at the concentrations specified by the physician. The acceptance test limits can also be defined according to the physician's specifications. The process consists of multiple rinses including reverse ultrafiltration, a bleach cleaning step, and further rinses prior to a testing step, which is followed by filling with sterilant. When supplied with a computer and printer, the documentation that is generated automatically includes patient and dialyzer information and the results of the dialyzer testing. The device also prints labels for placing on each reprocessed dialyzer. An option includes a bar code reader to identify hemodialyzers. With the computer option, use statistics may be compiled by patient, by the particular type of dialyzer, or for the entire unit's performance. Seratronics also markets a device for preparation of a stored dialyzer for the next patient use, the DPS 4. Essentially this is an automated device for circulating fluid on the blood side, while dialyzing off the sterilant. It includes an internal spectrophotometer for measuring residual formaldehyde concentrations.

The ADR-22 automated dialyzer reprocessing device is manufactured by Texas Medical Devices of Houston, Texas. This is a four-station unit that automatically provides documentation. The process consists of a rinsing step, including reverse ultrafiltration, and a hydrogen peroxide cleaning step prior to the testing stage. The manufacturer states that the ADR-22 may use bleach or other cleaning agents instead of peroxide, and that sterilants other than formaldehyde and gluteraldehyde may be used. The device is equipped with a bar code reader for identifying the particular dialyzer and patient. The documentation includes the channel on which the device was reprocessed, the patient, and dialyzer code numbers, the number of uses, and the cell volume coefficient, as well as the leak test result. Dialyzers are automatically passed or failed based on the criteria of the leak test, but, with cell volume and KUF, the operator must provide a decision on acceptance or rejection. In a year's study with 22 patients, Billiouw and coworkers [21] were able to reprocess two types of CUPROPHAN® hollow-fiber dialyzers an average of 5.6 times using the ADR-22 device. With the fourth and seventh uses of dialyzers, no significant drop in leukocytes occurred.

The Lixivitron 2 is a four-station automated reprocessing device that includes automated documentation; it is manufactured by Harco Medical Electronic Devices of Irvine, California. The process utilized by the Lixivitron consists of several dialyzer rinse steps and a reverse ultrafiltration prior to a cleaning step utilizing bleach solution. An additional rinse occurs prior to the testing steps. The Lixivitron will pass or fail a given dialyzer based on the results of the fiber bundle volume test and the transmembrane pressure leak test.

Documentation automatically supplied by the Lixivitron includes patient identification, dialyzer identification, the station number on which it was processed, the test results on cell volume, KUF and pressure leak test, as well as the conclusion of the machine and whether that dialyzer passed or failed. The number of uses is also recorded, as well as the number of cycles when the machine repeats a cleaning cycle on a dialyzer, if the dialyzer fails the volume test. Statistics can also be generated by the Lixivitron on performance of the whole facility. For example, statistics could include the total number of dialyzers processed, the number passed, the number failed, the number that were rejected by operator, the net passed, and the net failed. Statistics can also be generated by dialyzer type, where the average number of uses is calculated and the number of each of these types of dialyzers in service is given. Similarly, other data can be compiled on a per patient basis if desired.

The Compudial KP-1 is manufactured by Computer Dialysis Systems of Boulder, Colorado. It is a 12-station automated hemodialyzer reprocessing device that includes automatic generation of documentation. Reprocessors are also offered with fewer stations from four through 12. The process includes a number of rinse steps as well as a reverse ultrafiltration step, an optional bleach cleaning step, and further rinses prior to testing. Testing includes hemoglobin detection, a leak test, an ultrafiltration test, and, as an option, a residual cell volume test. Each dialyzer used with the Compudial automated documentation system is identified by a dialyzer key that is unique for a given patient. The key carries information on the specific dialyzer that has been prescribed, and other patient identification information. If the KP-1 is supplied with a remote control unit and printer as well as other ancillary equipment, an extensive variety of statistics similar to those mentioned for the Lixivitron can be generated automatically, or by simple instructions.

The Belro Company of Brussels, Belgium, has recently developed an automated dialyzer reprocessing machine that has six stations for simultaneous use. The process consists of rinsing, a sodium hypochlorite cleaning procedure, followed by disinfection with formaldehyde solution, over a 20- to 25-min cycle time. The approach used by the developers of this device also provides for the machine to function as an automated rinsing device to help prepare the hemodialyzers for the next use. Ultrafiltration characteristics of the hemodialyzers are tested in each case to determine whether the hemodialyzer is satisfactory. The Belro device functions in conjunction with an Apple computer to provide documentation of various elements, as well as the printing of labels.

A COMPARATIVE EVALUATION OF AUTOMATED REPROCESSING DEVICES

In view of the increased interest in hemodialyzer reprocessing, the greater utilization of automated techniques, and shortage of comparative data, a study was recently conducted to evaluate the devices commercially available in the US market [22, 23]. The scope included variability of test measures, relative changes of dialyzer properties, with number of uses and patient responses. A model of each of the devices was made available for evaluation at the Manhattan Kidney Center through the cooperation of the manufacturers. Devices included in the study were those described in table 11-1. Each was operated according to manufacturers' recommendations. Multistation devices were paired in a crossover study using 34 patients in two groups for an average of 182 treatments per study period. No crossover occurred in the study of single-station devices using 16 patients divided into two groups with an average of 122 treatments per period.

Study results with respect to reproducibility of test measures showed that, for multistation devices, the coefficient of variation (the standard deviation divided by the mean) for machine-measured dialyzer volumes was approximately 3%. The coefficient of variation of manually measured cell volumes performed in parallel with the machine measurements was 2%. For the single-station device tested, the coefficient was 1%. Coefficients of variation of machine measured ultrafiltration coefficients averaged about 2% with the exception of one device.

For evaluation of changes in dialyzer characteristics with use, machine and manually measured cell volumes and ultrafiltration coefficients were recorded. Prior to the first use, dialyzer characteristics were also measured. Mean values for each property together with standard deviations were calculated, and regression equations were generated for changes in properties with use for each device. The number of uses ranged from one through a maximum of 12 uses for each hemodialyzer. Hemodialyzers were arbitrarily removed from the study at the 12th use, but in a number of cases they may have been retired earlier.

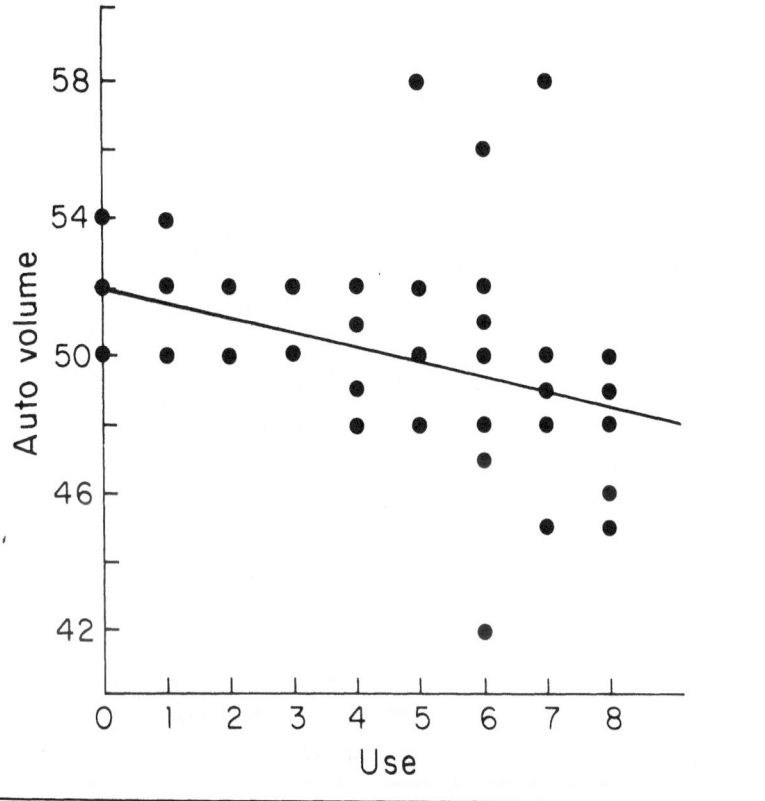

Figure 11-1. Changes in cell volume, measured on the Echo device, with use.

A sampling of data on dialyzer characteristics follows. In figure 11-1, the changes in cell volume, measured visually by the operator, versus hemodialyzer use, are shown for the Echo single-station reprocessing device. Individual data points are plotted in this figure. The regression equation for the automated volume vs use is: Automated volume = −0.433 (use) + 51.94, with an r value of −0.427. From the equation it is apparent that with 12 uses the cell volume has decreased approximately 10%.

The automated volume, determined by the Lixivitron device, as it changes with the number of uses is indicated in figure 11-2. The data plotted in this case represent the mean of merged data from two arms of the study that represents 20−25 individual data points from each of two groups of patients. The equation of the regression line is auto vol = −0.155 (use) + 51.452, with an r value of −0.849. With 12 uses the volume lost in this case is considerably below 10% of the original cell volume.

Automated volume and manual volume can correlate closely as shown in figure 11-3 using data from the Texas Medical ADR device. Individual data points are plotted and the regression equation is: auto vol = 1.45 (man vol)

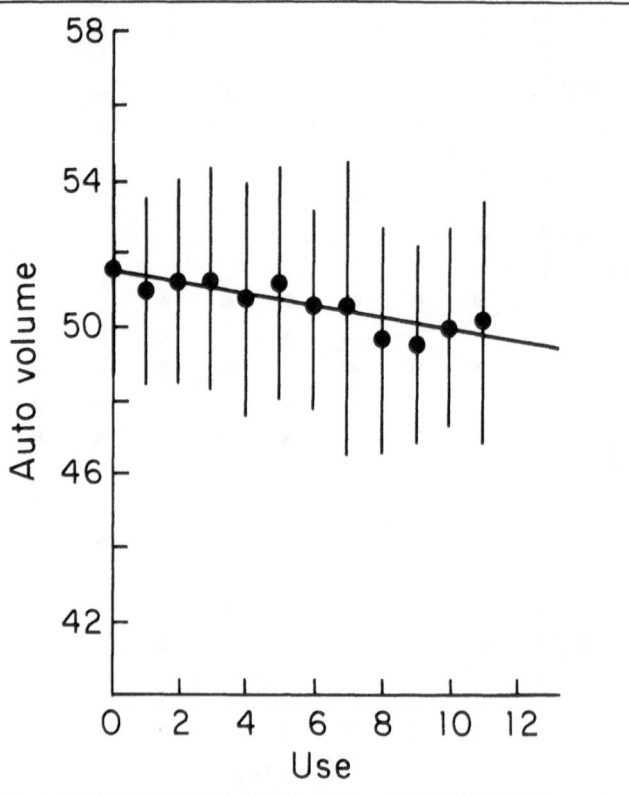

Figure 11-2. Changes in cell volume, measured on the LIXIVITRON® device, with use.

−27.863, with an r value of 0.98.

The plots in figure 11-4 show trends for each of six devices for changes in manual volume with use. The residual band of cell volumes decreased over 12 uses by a loss of approximately 4%−12%, depending on the machine.

In contrast to volume measurements, measurements of the ultrafiltration coefficient by machine varied over a wide range. The KUF may show increases or decreases with reuse. The reasons for the variation in KUF measurements were not investigated.

For further evaluation of the efficacy of reprocessing of hemodialyzers, a sample of the dialyzers that were removed from clinical service in the course of the study were subjected to in vitro measurements of urea and creatinine clearances as well as determinations of ultrafiltration coefficients. Relationships between these dialyzer characteristics and number of uses, dialyzer cell volume, and ultrafiltration coefficient were calculated. The clearance data were limited to the four multistation devices studied. Only those clearance values differing by less than 15% for blood and dialysate side clearances were selected. In figure 11-5 are shown data on urea and creatinine clearances

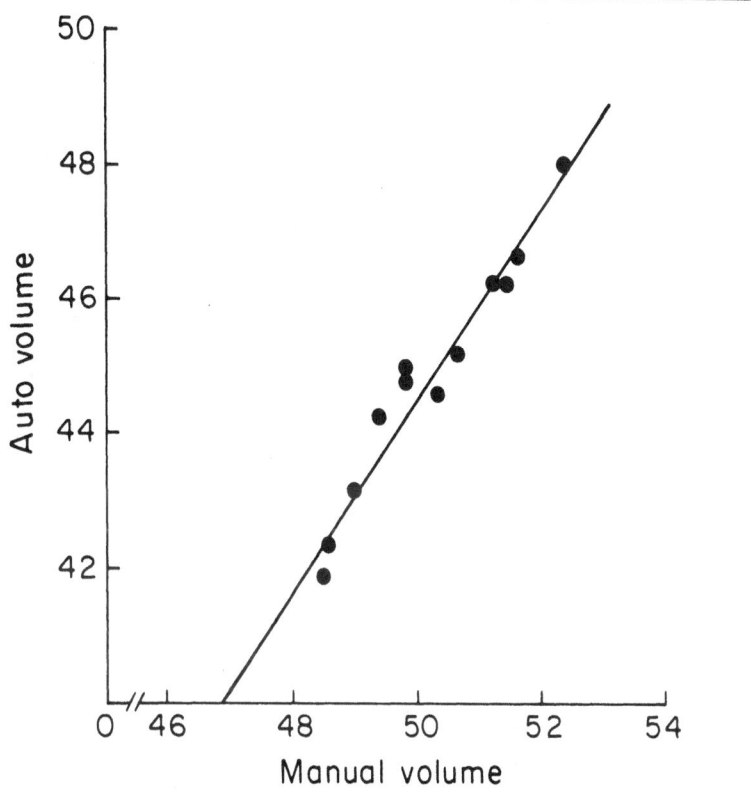

Figure 11-3. The regression line for cell volumes measured by the ADR® device, versus parallel manually measured volumes.

versus use. Regression equations are: urea clearance = 0.017 (use) + 152.8 (r = 0.005) and creatinine clearance = 0.223 (use) + 117.4 (r = 0.086). From the regression equations, it is clear that the clearance of urea and creatinine showed no correlation with use over the range of 12 uses studied. This result is consistent with the observed cell volume losses of 12% or less, for which, other experience has shown, there is no loss in clearance of small molecules such as urea and creatinine [24, 25].

During the in vitro measurements of clearance, ultrafiltration coefficients were determined (figure 11-6). The in vitro measured KUF showed a decrease of approximately 10% over the course of 12 uses. The regression equation is KUF = −0.024 (use) + 2.815 (r = −0.278).

Based upon the measures of physical properties and clearance characteristics of the reprocessed dialyzers, the machine reprocessed hemodialyzers are capable of providing essentially equivalent therapy to that provided by a new dialyzer within limits of approximately 10%.

Patient response to the hemodialyzers was measured by recording the

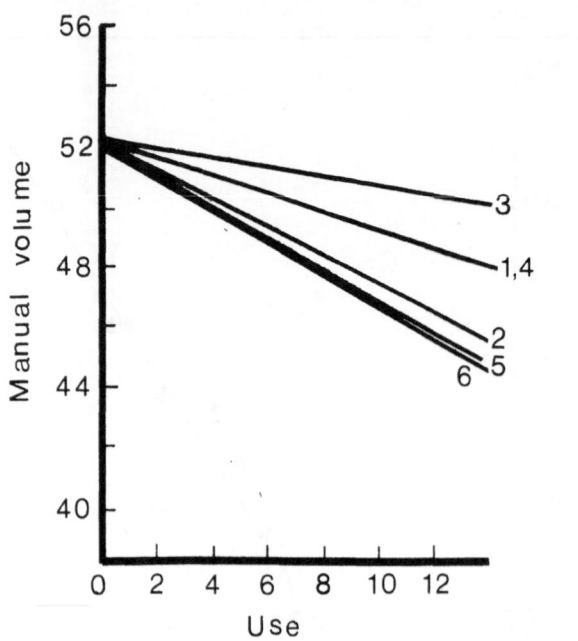

Figure 11-4. Changes in manually measured cell volumes with number of uses for all devices.

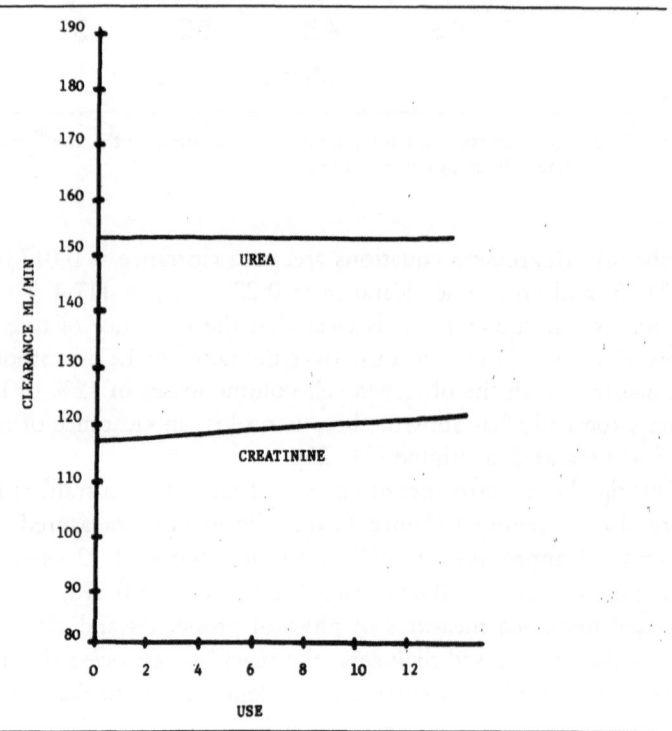

Figure 11-5. The lack of change in in vitro urea and creatinine clearance with use.

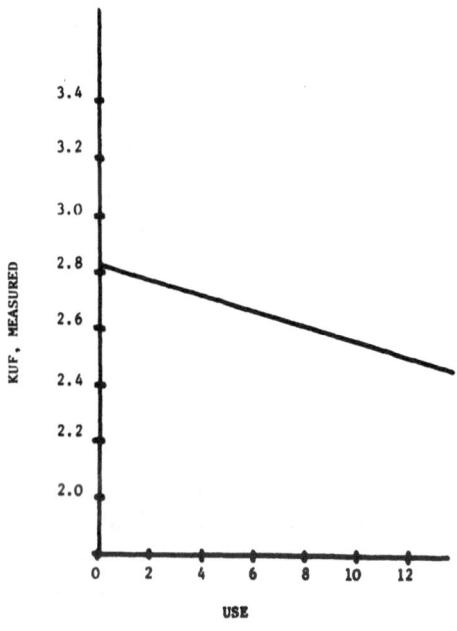

Figure 11-6. Changes in in vitro ultrafiltration coefficients with use.

intradialytic symptoms noted by the clinical staff in the treatment summaries. Intradialytic symptoms were tabulated into several categories and the incident rate per 100 treatments was calculated. The categories were back pain, cramps, nausea, pruritus, chest pain, fever or chill, dyspnea (shortness of breath), headache and other. The category nausea included nausea, vomiting, feeling ill, and dizziness. Cramps included cramps in any part of the body. Incidents of hyper- and hypotension were omitted since they were judged to be strongly operator influenced.

In addition to recording all complications and patient complaints or symptoms, intradialytic medications administered for treatment of such complaints or symptoms were also recorded. The most common medications were TYLENOL®, BENADRYL®, TEMARIL®, and DARVON®.

Intradialytic symptoms are summarized in table 11-2. The symptoms of back pain, fever/chill, dyspnea, headache, and other were combined and classified as other because the mean reprocessed device rate of these symptoms was less than 0.5 per 100 treatments. In table 11-2, AD A, AD B, etc., are notations for the various reprocessing devices; MRD represents the mean value for all reprocessing devices and NEW indicates the incidence for new hemodialyzers.

Nausea, which occurred at a mean rate of 5.2 for the reprocessed devices and 9.5 for new hemodialyzers, was the most common intradialytic symp-

Table 11-2. Intradialytic symptoms: events/100 treatments

Symptom	AD A	AD B	AD C	Reprocessing Device AD D	AD E	AD F	MRD	NEW
Cramps	3.1	1.8	5.3	4.9	1.7	2.4	2.8	4.1
Nausea	5.2	4.0	3.0	5.2	1.7	12.1	5.2	9.5
Pruritus	0.5	0.5	0.6	1.7	2.5	0	1.0	2.3
Chest pain	1.2	0.7	0	0.6	0.8	0.8	0.7	1.8
Other	1.0	2.7	0.6	4.1	0	3.2	2.0	8.4
Total	11.8	10.0	9.8	16.3	6.7	18.5	12.2	26.0
Medications	5.6	6.2	3.6	4.6	10.8	0.8	5.3	8.3

tom. The second most common symptom, cramps, occurred with a mean of
2.8 for the reprocessed devices compared with 4.1 events per 100 treatments
for new hemodialyzers. Pruritus was the third most common symptom,
occurring at a rate of one incident per 100 for the reprocessed devices
compared with 2.3 for new hemodialyzers. The total incidence of intradialytic symptoms recorded for the reprocessed devices was 12.2 per 100 treatments compared with 26 for new hemodialyzers.

The rate of usage of medications for intradialytic symptoms varied from a
low of 0.8 medications issued per 100 treatments to a high of 10.8 for the
reprocessing devices with a mean of 5.3. This compares with a usage of 8.3
medications per 100 treatments for new hemodialyzers.

The data were also examined to see how the rate of intradialytic symptoms
varied between the first quarter of reuses compared with the second, third,
and fourth. The result of this analysis is given in figure 11-7, which shows
the incidents per 100 treatments versus the treatment interval in the various
quarters. The average new dialyzer rate of 26 is shown as the top dotted line
in the figure with the reprocessed average rate of 12.2 as the lower line in the
figure. The closed circles represent the successive quarterly treatment average
rates, which decreased from 14.1 in the first quarter to 9.7 for uses ten
through 12 (fourth quarter). Intradialytic medication usage tended to confirm
this trend.

Judging from intradialytic patient response, all devices provided reprocessed hemodialyzers that showed biocompatibility equal or superior to that of
new hemodialyzers. The relative biocompatibility of a reprocessed dialyzer is
dependent on the characteristics of the new device, the specific process and
reagents employed [21], not on the nature of the automation. More extensive
research on this topic is in order (see chapter 2).

Utilization of automated processes has not eliminated or lessened the need
for strict quality control and quality assurance in a dialyzer reprocessing
program (see chapter 5). The specific tasks to be performed, calibrations to
be made, confirmations of chemical identities, concentration measures, etc.,
are different if an automated procedure is employed. Since any given center's

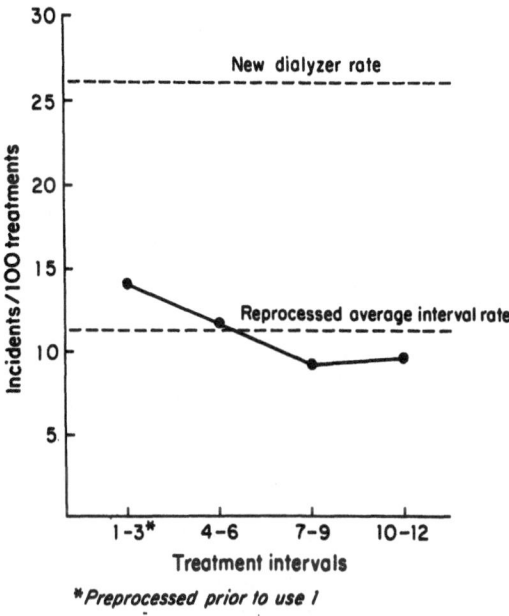

Figure 11-7. Trends in the incidence rate of intradialytic symptoms with quarterly intervals of reuse. Reprinted with the permission of the publisher from Trans Am Soc Artif Intern Organs 30:498-501, 1984.

program, procedures and equipment are unique, quality control and assurance require a detailed individualized analysis of potential failure modes, check points, etc. Although record keeping with automated machines is easier to accomplish than with strictly manual methods, other needs for calibrations, audits, etc., continue as with a manual system.

In summary, multiple factors should be examined. In table 11-3 are listed some factors for consideration in the choice of manual versus automated procedures or in selecting a particular reprocessing device. This decision is a very individual matter for each dialysis facility and requires an in-depth analysis of a variety of factors.

Table 11-3. Factors for consideration in selection of a reprocessing device or method

1. Indviduality of needs
2. Manual versus automated considerations
3. Personnel requirements
4. Changes in quality control
5. Interaction of patient schedules
6. Treated water demands
7. Supervisory needs
8. Maintenance requirements
9. Considerations of hybrid approaches
10. Environmental interactions

ACKNOWLEDGMENTS

The author wishes to express thanks to the manufacturers of the devices for their cooperation in providing them to the Manhattan Kidney Center for evaluation. Additionally, the author wishes to express appreciation to the following members of the Manhattan Kidney Center staff who provided technical assistance in the study: Phillip Andrysiak, James P. Burke, David Florin, Sandy Hu, Katherine Ling, Mary Liu, Brian Miller, William Miller, George Pace, David Stansfield, and Jenny Tsou.

REFERENCES

1. Shaldon SH, Dilva H, Rosen SM: Technique for refrigerated coil preservation haemodialysis with femoral venous catheterization. Br Med J 2:411–413, 1964.
2. Pollard TL, Barnett BMS, Eschbach JW, Scribner BH: A technique for storage and multiple reuse of the Kiil dialyzer and blood tubing. Trans Am Soc Artif Intern Organs 13:24–28, 1967.
3. DePalma JR, Mason B, Abykurah A: New artificial kidney reuse machine. Trans Am Soc Artif Intern Organs 20:584–588, 1974.
4. Ahmad R, Goldsmith HJ: Automated dialyzer rinsing machine. Dial Transplant 4(5):29 and 75, 1975.
5. Hardy DW, Higgins MR, McFarlane DF, Hughes RV: An automated cleaning device for dialyzers: machine design and technology. Clin Nephrol 5:276–278, 1976.
6. Deane N, Bemis JA: Multiple use of hemodialyzers. National Nephrology Foundation, New York, 1982.
7. Deane N: A survey of dialyzer reuse practice in the United States 1984. In: Hemodialyzer reuse: issues and solutions. Association for Advancement of Medical Instrumentation, Arlington VA, 1985, pp 1–5.
8. Alberttazzi A, Ruggeri G, Ardizzoia B, Franchini L, Burzi L: Automatic machine for dialyzer reuse. Proc Eur Dial Transplant Assoc 1:187–191, 1974.
9. Higgins MR, Grace M, Hardy DW, Silverberg DS: Clinical evaluation of an automated cleaning device for dialyzers. Clin Nephrol 5:251–255, 1976.
10. Vandenbroucke JM, Stragier A, Van Ypersele de Strihou C: Efficiency of automated reuse of disposable dialyzers. Proc Eur Dial Transplant Assoc 14:598–600, 1977.
11. Fitzcharles N, Elliot HL, McDougall AI: Clinical evaluation of an automated system for dialyzer reuse. Dial Transplant 9:825–828, 1980.
12. Man NK, Glace M, Becker A, Di Guilio S, Zingraff J, Funck-Brentano JL: A new dialyzer reuse machine. In: Frost TH (ed) Technical aspects of renal dialysis. Pitman, New York, 1978, pp 73–79.
13. Man NK, Lebkiri B, Polo P, De Sainte-Lorette E, Lemaire A, Funck-Brentano JL: Prevention of anti-N-like antibodies development with non-formaldehyde reuse procedure. Proc Dial Transplant Forum 10:18–21, 1980.
14. Lewis KJ, Ward MK, Kerr DNS: Residual formaldehyde in dialyzers: quantity, locations, and the effect of different methods of rinsing. Artif Organs 5:269–277, 1981.
15. Gentles W, Braganza LF, Saiphoo CS, Manuel MA: Programmable machine for dialyzer reuse. Med Biol Eng Comput 18:765–771, 1980.
16. Manuel MA, Saiphoo CS, Gentles W, Braganza LF: Clinical evaluation of a programmable machine for dialyzer reuse. Dial Transplant 11:206–211, 1982.
17. Bauer H, Brunner H, Franz HE: Experience with the disinfectant peroxyacetic acid (PES) for hemodialyzer reuse. Trans Am Soc Artif Intern Organs 29:662–665, 1983.
18. Hoenich NA, Johnson SRD, Buckley P, Harden J, Ward MK, Kerr DNS: Haemodialyzer reuse: impact on function and biocompatibility. Int J Artif Organs 6:261–266, 1983.
19. Gagnon RF, Kaye M: Hemodialysis neutropenia and dialyzer reuse: role of the cleansing agent. Uremia Invest 8:17–23, 1984.
20. Ogden DA, Friedl MM: Simultaneous reprocessing of hollow fiber dialyzers and blood tubing sets for multiple use. Dial Transplant 13:366–375, 1984.

21. Billiouw JM, Vanholder R, Piron M, Veirman R, Ringoir: Automated reuse of capillary hemodialyzers. Int J Artif Organs 8:83–88, 1985.
22. Deane N, Wineman RJ: Comparative evaluation of automated devices for reprocessing hemodialyzers: intradialytic patient response. Trans Am Soc Artif Intern Organs 30:498–501, 1984.
23. Wineman RJ: New technologies in automated reprocessing of hemodialyzers. In: Hemodialyzer reuse: issues and solutions. Association for Advancement of Medical Instrumentation, Arlington VA, 1985, pp 50–55.
24. Gotch F: Mass transport in reused dialyzers. Proc Dial Transplant Forum 10:81–86, 1980.
25. Gotch F: Correlation of transport properties with total cell volume (TCV) of new and reused hollow fiber dialyzers. In: Deane N, Bemis JA (eds) Multiple use of hemodialyzers. Final Report to the National Institute of Arthritis, Diabetes and Digestive and Kidney Diseases, Contract NO1-AM-9-2214, 1981, pp 53–64.

12. REGULATIONS AND STANDARDS

RONALD E. EASTERLING

A number of groups have published their positions on reuse of hemodialyzers and concerned physicians, nurses, technicians, and patients have developed advisory guidelines to promote safe and effective reprocessing methods. Some patients have complained of situations where they perceived evidence of improper reuse techniques (P. Lundin, personal communication). A representative of the National Association for Patients on Hemodialysis and Transplant (NAPHT) has urged external controls on the grounds that vested interests may undermine the medical profession's concern for the welfare of the patients (M. Klavins, unpublished). Certain governmental bodies agree that mandatory regulations on reuse of hemodialyzers are required to assure the public health and have promulgated mandatory standards. This chapter presents a general discussion of regulatory and standards activities followed by an analysis of the specific provisions of proposed and finalized regulations and standards (table 12-1).

GOVERNMENT ACTIVITIES

US federal government

The Health Care Financing Administration (HCFA) is responsible for the reimbursement and quality assurance of hemodialysis. The final rules for reimbursement of dialysis promulgated by the HCFA [1] state that

The ESRD community is currently divided on the issue of whether it is safe to reuse

Deane, Wineman, and Bemis (eds.): GUIDE TO REPROCESSING OF HEMODIALYZERS.
© 1986. Martinus Nijhoff Publishing. All rights reserved.

dialyzers which is one way a facility can reduce per treatment costs. In the notice of the proposed rule making, we explained that we were neutral on this issue. We are neither supporting or prohibiting it in these final regulations.

The final rules go on to indicate that the HCFA will continue to monitor the outcomes of facilities that reuse to determine whether the rules should be changed from the standpoint of health and safety or reimbursement with respect to reuse.

Since reuse of dialyzers is "one way of reducing treatment costs," facilities that do reuse dialyzers have lower supply costs than those that use only new dialyzers, producing a financial incentive for reuse. In fact, some facilities have elected to begin reuse to make ends meet under the prospective rate. This has heightened concern about quality control and quality assurance for the reprocessing procedure.

The HCFA has "networks" composed of representatives of the facilities in the region that are charged with conducting activities designed to evaluate the quality of care and to maintain an acceptable level of the quality of care. An informal survey of the 32 networks yielded ten responses. One network has taken no action on this issue. One network endorses the Revised Standards for Reuse of Hemodialyzers of the National Kidney Foundation [2]. Five have developed documents on reuse of hemodialyzers varying from a position statement with general requirements that are subject to review by the Medical Review Board to detailed recommendations. None of these endorses or prohibits the practice of reprocessing dialyzers. This is consistent with the statement from the Office of Coverage Policy, Bureau of Eligibility, Reimbursement and Coverage in August 1984 that it is premature to consider a change in the regulations from the standpoint of reuse of hemodialyzers (R.A. Steimer, personal communication). The seven specific guidelines that have been developed by the network coordinating councils (NCC) are discussed in the final section of this chapter.

The Center for Devices and Radiological Health (CDRH) of the Food and Drug Administration (FDA) has the responsibility of implementing the Medical Device Amendments of 1976 to the Food, Drug and Cosmetic Act. The following discussion is largely based on a paper presented by the chairman of the reuse committee of the CDRH (L. Kobren, unpublished). The statute requires the FDA to see that products entering the marketplace are safe and effective. Additionally, the FDA has a more general mission to protect the public health, which may be done by nonregulatory means. As part of this activity, a Compliance Policy Guideline was issued on reuse of disposable medical devices that states [3]:

The institution or practitioner who reuses a disposable medical device should be able to demonstrate that: (1) the device can be adequately cleansed and sterilized, (2) physical characteristics or quality of the device will not be adversely affected, and, (3)

185

the device remains safe and effective for its intended use. Moreover, since disposable devices are not intended by the manufacturer or the distributor for reuse, any institution or practitioner who resterilizes and/or reuses a disposable medical device must bear full responsibility for its safety and effectiveness. Additionally, FDA requests that any information developed regarding this practice should be referred to the Center for Devices and Radiological Health for review and evaluation. The Center will determine if adverse effects resulting from the procedure was a user problem or was related to improper labeling.

The statement "For Single Use Only" on the label of hemodialyzers is not required by the FDA. Manufacturers are required to provide the user with adequate directions for use, and they have thus far maintained that, since they cannot be sure a user would follow directions for reprocessing, they cannot assume the liability implicit in instructions for reuse. If a manufacturer were to apply for a hemodialyzer labeled for reuse, the application probably would be considered. While the CDRH authorized marketing of automated hemodialyzer reprocessing machines, the basis for this determination is that these devices are substantially equivalent to devices marketed prior to the Medical Device Amendments of 1976. Hence the CDRH did not consider the merits of reuse of hemodialyzers in making this decision. The labeling was reviewed, which includes a statement that, while the device reprocesses the hemodialyzer, the physician is solely responsible for the safety and effectiveness of the device. A recent legal opinion that the FDA does not have the authority to require manufacturers to label disposable devices for reuse is under study. Nevertheless, the FDA, in concert with other members of the medical community, is attempting to persuade manufacturers to voluntarily include labeling information useful to those who reprocess devices such as certain information on material properties of the device. In any event, if the FDA finds that the public health is at risk due to reuse of dialyzers, action will be taken. Possible approaches include education, publicity, and other nonregulatory actions. Furthermore, contacts have been instituted with several state health departments to identify areas that may require regulatory action. Reuse procedures are among the items that will be reviewed in this effort. A possible outcome of this activity is promulgation of quality assurance programs similar to those already in place in the medical radiology area. In the meantime, the CDRH is working with the Association for Advancement of Medical Instrumentation (AAMI) in its effort to develop guidelines for reuse of hemodialyzers (this is a voluntary recommended practice as described later in this chapter).

State governments

Increasingly, state governments have become involved in regulating reuse of hemodialyzers. The following discussion may be incomplete or inaccurate, since a survey of specific regulations by state governments is not available, and there may be proposed regulations in other states or the material presented here may be out of date. In view of the growing promulgation of state regulations, it is important to check on local regulations when instituting a dialyzer reprocessing program. The state department of health or other licensing agency, the ESRD network coordinating council, and facilities reprocessing dialyzers in the region are likely sources of pertinent information.

In 1981, the Alabama State Committee on Public Health, Board of Health, banned reuse of any one-time-use disposable item. In 1982, hemodialyzers were exempt from this prohibition, and facilities were asked to submit their protocol. The Licensure Division of the Bureau of Licensure and Certification, Department of Public Health, visits facilities to ensure that the facility's protocol is being followed. However, requirements for reuse protocols have not been established by the Department of Public Health [4].

In 1981, the Colorado Department of Health prohibited reuse of medical devices labeled as single use or disposable with the exception of hemodialyzers [5]. Specific requirements were established for reuse of hemodialyzers ("dialyzer regeneration"). Highlights of these regulations are given later and in table 12-1.

A California law finalized in 1981 requires the State Department of Public Health to establish a protocol for reuse of hemodialyzers. As of early 1984, hearings on the proposed regulations were still in progress [6]. The proposed hemodialyzer regulations from 1983 are summarized in the last section and in table 12-1. These contain a statement that deviation from any of the provisions without an alternative reuse protocol approved by the Department constitutes a violation of the Health and Safety Code.

In 1984, the Illinois Hospital Licensing Board proposed to change hospital licensing requirements to prohibit "processing and reuse of single patient use supplies." The adoption of this proposed change has been delayed [7]. In the meantime, ESRD Network Council 15 has adopted guidelines for dialyzer reuse in preparation since 1982.

In 1984, New Mexico developed proposed regulations for out-patient dialysis facilities that include requirements for reuse of hemodialyzers. These requirements are summarized in table 12-1 and the last section of the chapter.

A survey of state authorities conducted by the Alabama Department of Health in 1981 yielded 47 responses [8]. Thirteen states have licensure laws for ESRD facilities. In five of these states, the law addressed reuse of hemodialyzers and, in four of them, this practice is permitted. None of the 34 states that do not license ESRD facilities had laws that prohibit reuse of hemodialyzers.

JOINT COMMISSION ON THE ACCREDITATION OF HOSPITALS (JCAH)

In 1983, the JCAH standard on reuse stated: "There shall be written guidelines for the storage, handling, use and disposition of disposable items.

Disposable items should not be reused" [9]. A nurse surveyor and field representative for the JCAH reported that this statement would not necessarily jeopardize a hospital's accreditation [10]. The information submitted by a reviewer is evaluated by the joint commission that, in the final analysis, is concerned with the quality of care. If action were taken, the institution "would most likely receive a contingency under the present three-year cycle, meaning that the facility would have to either submit in writing answers to questions submitted by the commissioners or to receive a focus survey (within six months) for the area found deficient." It was observed in the preface to the proceedings of this conference that "attempts should be made to persuade the commission that it is reasonable to change this criterion to accept reuse if proper protocols are followed and documented" [11]. The author is unaware of any action taken on this matter or any instance where accreditation by the JCAH has been threatened because of the reuse of hemodialyzers.

VOLUNTARY STANDARDS DEVELOPMENT

In 1982, the National Kidney Foundation published standards for reuse of hemodialyzers developed by "representatives of the voluntary and scientific members of the foundation" [12], and these standards were revised in 1983 by "a group of physicians, nurses, consumers (patients), industry representatives and microbiologists" [3]. These standards (RS-NKF) are summarized subsequently and in table 12-1.

In 1982, the Dialysis Technical Subcommittee of the Health Industry Manufacturers Association (HIMA) prepared a statement on reuse of hemodialyzers [13] in response to the report on reuse of hemodialyzers by Deane and Bemis to the National Institutes of Health [14]. The HIMA points out that using formaldehyde as a germicide results in disinfection rather than sterilization that is required by the FDA for new dialyzers, calls attention to the possible environmental hazards of reuse procedures, asserts that the tests for biocompatibility and nonpyrogenicity conducted on new dialyzers were not addressed, suggests that the potential for hazards may be increased because process control methods may not be as thorough as those used by manufacturers, states that the liability for patient injury results from failing to follow the manufacturer's instructions and warnings, and proposes that the cost savings from reuse may be reduced if all costs for remanufacturing a dialyzer to the same quality levels as a new dialyzer are considered.

In 1983, the AAMI convened a technology assessment conference on reuse of disposables. The scope of this meeting included all disposables, but many of the presentations addressed reuse of hemodialyzers. Position statements were given by several organizations [15]. The Association of Practitioners in Infection Control felt that it would be short-sighted to categorically endorse or oppose reuse of disposables. The ECRI (formerly the Emergency Care Research Institute) recommended national guidelines of general scope, de-

Table 12-1. Comparison of standards and regulations (see text)

AAMI proposed recommended practice	Standards								Regulations		
		Networks									
	NKF[a]	5[b]	14[b]	15[b]	19[b]	25[b]	27[b]	32[b]	CO[c]	CA[d]	NM[e]
Records											
Master	–	–	–	–	–	–	–	–	–	–	–
Reprocessing	+	+	+	+	–	+	+	+	+	+	+
Equipment maintenance	–	–	–	–	–	–	–	–	–	+	–
Material quality	–	–	–	–	–	–	–	–	–	–	–
Complaint investigation	+	–	+	–	–	+	+	–	+	+	–
QA and QC[f]	+	–	+	+	–	+	+	+	+	+	–
Personnel											
Qualifications	–	–	+	+	–	–	–	+	–	+	–
Curriculum	+	–	+	+	–	+	+	+	+	+	+
Documentation	+	+	+	+	–	+	–	+	+	+	+
Medical issues											
Indications	–	–	–	–	–	–	–	–	–	–	–
Contraindications	+	–	+	+	+	+	+	+	+	+	–
Hepatitis	–	–	+	+	+	+	+	+	+	+	–
Other[g]	+	+	+	+	+	–	–	–	+	+	+
Informed consent	+	+	+	+	–	–	+	+	+	+	+
Equipment											
Water systems	–	–	–	+	–	–	–	+	+	–	–
Reprocessing equipment	–	–	–		–	–	–	–	–	–	–
Environmental control equipment	–	–	+		–	–	–	–	–	–	–
Safety equipment	+	–	+		–	+	+	–	–	+	–
Physical Plant											
Reprocessing area	+	–	+	+	–	+	+	–	+	+	–
Storage area	–	+	+	+	–	–	–	–	+	+	–
Laboratory area	–	–	–	–	–	–	–	–	–	–	–

	C1	C2	C3	C4	C5	C6	C7	C8	C9	C10	C11
Personnel protection	+	−	+	+	+	+	−	+	+	+	+
Environmental safety	−	+	+	+	+	+	−	+	+	+	+
Reprocessing supplies	−	−	−	−	−	−	−	−	−	−	−
Hemodialyzer labelling											
Time of labeling	−	+	−	+	−	+	−	−	+	+	−
Label composition	−	+	−		−	+	−	+	+		+
Information recorded	−	+	+		+	+	−	+	+		+
Termination of dialysis											
Rinsing/cleaning											
Timing	−	+	−	−	−	−		+	−		−
Rinsing/cleaning agents	+	+	+	+	+	+	+	−	+	+	+
Interfacing components	−	+	−	+	−	−		+	+		−
Visual result	−	−	+	−	−	+	+	+	−	+	+
Performance measurements											
Clearance											
Test after each use	+	+	+	+	+	+		+	+		+
HFAK (FBV)	+	+	+	+	+	+		+	+		+
Other	−	+	−	−	−	+		+	−		−
Validation											
Ultrafiltration rate											
in vivo	−	−	−	−	−	−		−	−		−
in vitro	−	+	−	−	−	−		−	−		+
Blood integrity test	−	−	+	+	−	−	+	+	−	+	+
Disinfection/sterilization											
Interior											
Germicide											
Reagent	+	+	+	−	+	+		+	+		+
Formaldehyde	+	+	+	−	+	+		+	+	+	+
Other	−	+	−	−	+	+		+	+		−
Diluent for germicide	−	+	−	+	−	+		+	+		−
Monitoring	−	+	−	+	−	−	−	−	+		−
Exterior											
Inspection	−	−	+	−	+	+		+	+	−	+
Disposition of rejects	−	−	−	−	−	−		−	+	−	−

Table 12-1. continued

AAMI proposed recommended practice	NKF[a]	Networks							Regulations		
		5[b]	14[b]	15[b]	19[b]	25[b]	27[b]	32[b]	CO[c]	CA[d]	NM[e]
Preparation for dialysis											
Inspection	+	–	–	+	–	+	–	–	+	–	–
Patient identification	+	+	+	+	+	+	+	+	+	–	–
Presence of germicide	+	–	+	–	+	–	–	–	+	–	+
Residual potentially toxic substances	+	–	+	+	+	+	+	+	+	+	+
Time of exposure to germicide	–	–	–	+	–	+	–	–	–	–	–
Monitoring during dialysis											
Symptoms/signs	+	+	+	+	–	+	+	–	+	+	+
Dialyzer failures	+	–	–	+	–	+	+	–	+	+	–
QA and QC procedures[h]	+	–	–	+	–	+	+	+	–	+	–

[a] National Kidney Foundation Revised Standards for Reuse of Hemodialyzers [3].
[b] ESRD Network Coordinating Council Numbers.
[c] Colorado Department of Public Health (proposed revision of 1981 regulation — the facility must submit a protocol that meets the guidelines in the regulation).
[d] Proposed Regulations of the California Department of Public Health (alternative proposals can be submittd for review).
[e] Regulations Governing Renal Dialysis Outpatient Facility Licensing, New Mexico Health and Environment Department Health Services Division.
[f] QA, quality assurance; and QC, quality control.
[g] AIDS and septicemia.
[h] The Proposed AAMI Recommended Practice states that there is a difference of opinion as to whether specific informed consent for reuse is appropriate, while a *plus* (+) in the table means that specific informed consent is recommended or required.

signation of the number of reuses that are safe, and sharing of knowledge on reuse by manufacturers. The International Association of Hospital Service Management recognized that some items are reusable and some are not, and urged manufacturers/to provide protocols for reuse when appropriate. The American College of Legal Medicine recommended that protocols on reuse be supplied by manufacturers and that physicians should obtain informed consent for reuse. The American Society for Artificial Internal Organs favored reuse of hemodialyzers as long as safe, effective protocols are used, believed that the physician is responsible for reuse of hemodialyzers, considered clinically proven methods not to be investigational, and believed that informed consent for reuse may be included in the overall consent form for hemodialysis. The NAPHT felt that patients want assurance that reuse is in their best interests and advocated further research on the safety and adequacy of reused dialyzers. The Renal Physicians Association believed that reuse of hemodialyzers is done on the prescription of the physician and noted the position of the HCFA on reuse of hemodialyzers (see above). The National Kidney Foundation recognized that potentially toxic substances can be reduced by appropriate procedures to the point that acute reactions to new and used dialyzers are infrequent and that chronic toxicity has not been described. Additionally it was felt that the growing practice of reuse now makes it mandatory to develop standards of safety and performance for reprocessed dialyzers (the 1982 version of the standards developed by the foundation are also given verbatim; see the last section and table 12-1 for the 1983 revised standards).

In December of 1983, the AAMI authorized the Reuse Subcommittee of the Renal Disease and Detoxification Committee, consisting of representatives of the CDRH, the Centers for Disease Control, the American Society for Artificial Internal Organs, the AAMI, the American Nephrology Nurses Association, the NAPHT, the National Kidney Foundation, and the HIMA, as well as individual physicians and manufacturer representatives who volunteered their services. To develop a recommended practice for reuse of dialyzers, the resulting draft of the AAMI Recommended Practice for Reuse of Hemodialyzers was the subject of a technology assessment conference in November 1984. Balloting on the document is expected in 1985. Once it has achieved a consensus of the committee, it will be subjected to national review. The final recommended practice will be updated as necessary (AAMI policy requires review at least every five years).

An AAMI recommended practice is a consensus document that is not intended to be applicable in all situations. Nevertheless, these documents are well known in governmental and legal circles, so the practitioner must be prepared to defend deviations from the standards.

The AAMI also develops standards addressed to the manufacturer. These documents are called "standards" rather than "recommended practices." In the case of reuse of hemodialyzers, a standard could be developed for equipment marketed to reprocess hemodialyzers.

SPECIFIC PROVISIONS OF REGULATIONS AND STANDARDS (1984)

Table 12-1 compares the topics discussed in the Proposed AAMI Recommended Practice for Reuse of Hemodialyzers (AAMI-RP), the Revised Standards for Reuse of Hemodialyzers of the National Kidney Foundation (RS-NKF), guidelines developed by the ESRD network councils, and the state regulations. The following discussion is not a substitute for review of the actual documents, which are more detailed and subject to change. It is intended only to highlight major issues and give an idea of the range of approaches.

A *plus* (+) in the table means that the topic is addressed and a *minus* (−) indicates that it is not. When a main category is covered in general terms but the subtopics of the AAMI-RP are not addressed specifically, a *plus* is recorded for the main topic of the other document and the subtitle entries are left blank. With the exception of informed consent, the topics listed for the AAMI-RP contain specific recommendations and a *plus* for another document means that the document also has a specific recommendation or requirement. On the contrary, the section on informed consent in the AAMI-RP presents the controversy about the appropriateness of specific informed consent for reuse of hemodialyzers while a *plus* for another standard or a regulation means that informed consent is recommended or required.

Since the AAMI-RP is a voluntary consensus document that may not be applicable in all cases, it is not surprising that its scope is broader than mandatory regulations, which are addressed to qualified medical practitioners. Additionally, it specifically addresses matters that may be implied by other recommendations or requirements. For example, a requirement to control environmental pollutants implies operation and maintenance of equipment that is not discussed in other documents. These sections are included in the AAMI-RP to asssist the personnel in charge of reuse programs who often have limited expertise in this area.

The records section of the AAMI-RP recommends the types of files to document the reuse procedure and various quality assurance (QA) and quality control (QC) activities. These files are frequently implied by the other documents, but generally are not specifically addressed.

The AAMI-RP outlines a recommended curriculum for personnel doing reuse of hemodialyzers that is more detailed than the material addressing curriculum in the other documents. Several categories of qualification are mentioned in the AAMI-RP that are not covered in the other documents.

Unlike the other documents, the AAMI-RP includes a section on indications for reuse, e.g., first-use syndrome and improvement of the quality of care or access to dialysis resulting from reuse. The contraindications are infectious diseases that may be contracted by the staff or that increase the microbial contamination of the dialyzer, as well as hypersensitivity to the reagents used to reprocess the dialyzer. Nearly all the documents list hepatitis as a contraindication for reuse. The data showing no more hepatitis in staff working in facilities that reuse compared with those working in units that do not [16] cannot be considered support for reuse of hemodialyzers used by patients with hepatitis B since most units have taken the a priori position that hemodialyzers used by patients with hepatitis B should not be reused. One document recognizes the possibility of reusing hepatitis-B-positive dialyzers in areas isolated for this disease.

Nearly all documents require or recommend separate informed consent by the patient for reuse of his or her hemodialyzer. The AAMI-RP does not make a recommendation on this issue. Instead it describes the controversy about whether reuse of the hemodialyzer should be singled out from other aspects of the hemodialysis procedure for specific informed consent. A representative of the NAPHT recently reiterated the position of this organization that there should be specific informed consent for reuse of the hemodialyzer (M. Klavins, personal communication).

The equipment section of the AAMI-RP is largely performance oriented and includes suggested maintenance and validation procedures. References to equipment in the other documents are more general with the exception of safety equipment and, in some cases, submicron filtration of water used for reuse. The AAMI-RP compares manual and automated systems in general terms. This topic is not mentioned by the other documents.

The physical plant section of the AAMI-RP allows for reprocessing in the patient area under certain conditions, unlike the other documents that address this issue. The material in AAMI-RP on ventilation, design characteristics, laboratory area, and environmental safety is implied by a number of other documents, but none deal with these matters in detail with the exception of the Colorado regulations. This document requires that, if general ventilation is used, the exhaust vent should be less than 6 inches above the floor because formaldehyde is heavier than air. While this stipulation implies that formaldehyde is the only germicide used, the possibility of other germicides is recognized elsewhere. A number of documents directly address the storage area and personnel protection.

The AAMI-RP deals with specifications for materials in general terms as well as incoming supply control and inventory control. This area is not covered by the other documents.

The section on hemodialyzer labeling in the AAMI-RP recommends the time of labeling relative to the first use, the characteristics of the label material, and the information that is considered a minimum for patient safety. The most common information required or recommended by the other documents is identification to ensure that reprocessed dialyzer is used only for the patient who used it the first time. There also is general agreement that the number of reuses should appear on the label. The AAMI-RP also mentions other information that could be included on the label. Several of the documents indicate that the label composition should resist defacement during reprocessing.

The reprocessing procedure is addressed by all of the documents although two only mention the need for cleaning/rinsing, performance testing, and disinfection/sterilization. Most of the documents recommend RO quality water for rinsing/cleaning and two recommend submicron filtration of the water used in reprocessing.

All of the documents specify a performance test for each dialyzer prior to reuse. The AAMI-RP recommends a urea clearance that is 90%−110% of the original value. Indirect tests are permitted and, in the case of hollow-fiber dialyzers, the corresponding fiber bundle volume (FBV) is recommended, noting that this value is usually 80% of the original FBV. The RS-NKF specifies a minimum FBV of 80% of the original value and states that only clearance tests can be used to monitor other types of dialyzers at the present time. Limits for clearance are not specified. The proposed California protocol specifies a minimum urea or creatinine clearance of 90% of the original value and a minimum vitamin B_{12} or inulin clearance of 80% of the original value. This criterion takes into account the differences between small and large molecule clearance. Suitably validated indirect tests are permitted and, in the case of hollow-fiber dialyzers, a minimum FBV is specified, e.g., 80% of the original value. The other documents fall within these guidelines, most often specifying a minimum FBV for hollow-fiber dialyzers that is 80% of the original value. There are two notable exceptions. The NCC 15 guideline recommends a minimim clearance (molecule not specified) of hollow-fiber FBV of 85% of the original value. Considering the difference between the clearance of small and large molecules (see proposed California protocol above), apparently the intent is that "clearance" includes vitamin B_{12} or inulin clearance. The New Mexico regulation also does not specify the test molecule for clearance, but permits a hollow-fiber dialyzer FBV of 80% of the original value. In this case the intent appears to be either that "clearance" is urea or creatinine clearance, or to set a less stringent standard for hollow-fiber dialyzers than for other types of dialyzers.

The ultrafitration performance test is controversial because of the difference between in vitro and in vivo results and the wide variation in the ultrafiltration characteristics of new dialyzers (the American National Standard for First Use Hemodialyzers, which is addressed to the manufacturer, recommends a ± 20% variation for the stated value because of the state of the art in membrane technology [17]). Accordingly, the NCC 15 recommendation that the ultrafiltration rate of the reprocessed dialyzer be within 15% of the manufacturer's reported values is inconsistent with the limits recommended for new dialyzers. In addition to monitoring the ultrafiltration rate to determine the efficacy of the dialyzer for removing fluid, ultrafiltration has also been recommended as an alternative test for monitoring clearance [18]. The accuracy of this approach has been challenged [19]. The rationale of the AAMI-RP discusses this issue. None of the other documents propose ultrafiltration as an alternative for clearance to monitor solute transport.

The initial Colorado regulation limits the number of reuses to eight. The most recent version of this document drops this restriction. If this deletion is adapted, Colorado will join the rest of the regulations and standards using performance as the criterion for rejection of a reprocessed dialyzer rather than an arbitrary number of reuses.

In view of the widespread use of formaldehyde as a germicide for reprocessed dialyzers, data on the concentration and exposure time for adequate disinfection of the dialyzer (and the potential for toxicity due to this agent) are reflected in specific recommendations or requirements concerning this substance in all but one of the documents that specifically address germicides. The AAMI-RP, RS-NKF, New Mexico regulations, and one of the NCC guidelines recommend or require at least 4% formaldehyde for a minimum of 24 h, while the proposed California protocol recommends at least 1.5% for a minimum of 36 h. The Colorado regulation specifies at least 2% for a minimum of 24 h. Most of the documents recognize that there may be other suitable germicides, but none specify concentrations or conditions for any of these.

The AAMI-RP and the RS-NKF recommend that the dilutent for the germicide should have a bacterial pyrogen level of less that 1 ng/ml (the published RS-NKF [3] has a typographical error, e.g., the level is given as 1 mg/ml rather than 1 ng/ml). The NCC 14 guidelines recommends that, in the event of a suspected pyrogenic reaction with reprocessed dialyzers, the water used for preparing the germicides should be checked for a bacteria lipopolysaccharide (pyrogen) level of less than 1 ng/ml by the limulus amoebocyte lysate assay or an equivalent test. The NCC 15 guidelines has a similar recommendation, but this document recommends that all of the water used for reprocessing meet this criterion. The AAMI-RP and the RS-NKF do not recommend routine cultures to monitor the disinfection/sterilization process while some of the other documents do.

The inspection requirements or recommendations specify a clear effluent. In the case of hollow-fiber dialyzers, small peripheral clots in the headers and a few dark fibers are allowed (the RS-NKF specifies fewer than five dark fibers).

All of the documents specify care to ensure that the patient is not dialyzed with dialyzer that has been used by another patient. A test for the presence of the germicide in the dialyzer before preparing the dialyzer for dialysis is specified by the AAMI-RP and several other documents. The maximum permissible level of formaldehyde in the effluent from the dialyzer is 5 ppm in all of the documents except the proposed California protocol, which uses the detection limit for formaldehyde, e.g., 1 ppm; 5 ppm is recommended in the AAMI-RP due to the lack of toxicity at this level and the difficulty encountered in lowering the level to 1 ppm, especially when 4% formaldehyde is used. No residual level is specified for the other germicides by any of the documents except to indicate that it should be safe.

All of the documents specify pre- and postdialysis body temperature measurements as a monitor of the reprocessing procedure. Additionally, the AAMI-RP covers other unexplained symptoms. Recording and analysis of dialyzer failures is recommended by the AAMI-RP and most of the other documents specify or imply this item.

The AAMI-RP details the frequency of quality assurance (QA — updating and implementation of written policies and protocols) and quality control (QC — validation tests) activities. This recommendation is not made or required by the other documents. It also recommends that the QA and QC person(s) should not be directly involved in the reprocessing procedure. Two of the other documents have similar recommendations.

The RS-NKF states that home dialysis patients should follow the same standards as the center and that the procedure should be reviewed semi-annually in the home setting. Two of the other documents have similar recommendations. The more comprehensive AAMI-RP exempts the home dialysis patient from provisions applicable only to the dialysis facility. The NCC 27 guideline specifies that, if reprocessing is done outside the facility, the facility is responsible for the procedure. The AAMI-RP does not address blood tubing reuse because a consensus on this issue could not be achieved at the present time. The proposed California regulations permit reuse of blood tubing when it is treated as an integral part of the dialyzer. None of the documents endorses or discourages reuse of hemodialyzers.

REFERENCES

1. Department of Health and Human Services, Health Care Financing Administration: Medicare program; end-stage renal disease program; prospective reimbursement for dialysis services and approval of special purpose facilities; final rule, 1983. Fed Register 48: 21272, 1983.
2. National Kidney Foundation: Revised standards for reuse of hemodialyzers, December 2, 1983. Contemp Dial 5(2):29 and 37, 1984.
3. Food Drug Administration (FDA): Compliance policy guide 7124.16: reuse of medical disposable devices, chapter 24, devices, July 1, 1981. Contemp Dial 3(6):32, 1982.
4. Alabama reverses itself and allows reuse. Contemp Dial 3(6):40, 1982.
5. Colorado Department of Public Health: 6C.C.R. 1011-1 chapter 11: Licensure, 7.0: single use of disposable medical devices. Contemp Dial 3(7):21, 1982.
6. California reuse delay continues. Contemp Dial 5(2):10, 1984.
7. Illinois reuse ban delayed. Contemp Dial 5(9):13, 1984.
8. Zom TS: Study of the reuse of renal dialyzers. Contemp Dial 3(10):34–40, 1982.
9. JCAH: Accreditation manual of hosptials. Joint Commission on the Accreditation of Hospitals, Chicago, 1983.
10. Barnes A: Reuse and JCAH accreditation. AAMI Technical Assessment Report 6-83: reuse of disposables. Association for the Advancement of Medical Instrumentation, Arlington VA, 1983.
11. Easterling RE: Introduction, commentary and direction for the future. AAMI Technical Assessment Report 6-83: reuse of disposables. Association for the Advancement of Medical Instrumentation, Arlington VA, 1983.

12. Ogden DA: If carefully observed, new National Kidney Foundation dialyzer reuse standards offer assurance of safe, effective dialysis. Contemp Dial 5(2):5, 1984.
13. Taylor JD: Dialyzer reuse: industry concerns regarding the practice or remanufacture and reuse of single-use hemodialyzers. Contemp Dial 3(7):52–56, 1982, and 3(8):47–50, 1982.
14. Deane N, Bemis JA: Multiple use of hemodialyzers: final report to the National Institute of Arthritis, Diabetes and Digestive and Kidney Diseases. Contract NO1-AM-9-2214. June 1981, pp 53–64.
15. Epilogue. AAMI Technical Assessment Report 6-83: reuse of disposables. Association for the Advancement of Medical Instrumentation, Arlington VA, 1983, pp 88–94.
16. Favero MS, Deane N, Leger RT, Sosin HE: Effect of multiple use of dialyzers on hepatitis B incidence in patients and staff. JAMA 245:166–167, 1981.
17. American National Standard for First Use Hemodialyzers. Association for the Advancement of Medical Instrumentation, Arlington VA, 1984.
18. Pizzaconi VB: QA and QC aspects of reuse. AAMI Technical Assessment Report 6-83: reuse of disposables. Association for the Advancement of Medical Instrumentation, Arlington VA, 1983, pp 76–82.
19. Gotch FA: Quality control tests for validation of dialyzer performance. AAMI Technical Assessment Report: hemodialyzer reuse: issues and solutions. Association for the Advancement of Medical Instrumentation, Arlington VA, 1985, pp 37–41.

INDEX

Definition of 64
Dialysis Delivery Systems 65
High-level 65
Low-level 65
Quality Control 65
DOCUMENTATION 77
DYLADE DS^R 113
DYSPNEA 117

ECRI (Emergency Care Research Institute) 187
EDTA, (EUROPEAN DIALYSIS AND TRANSPLANT ASSOCIATION) CLINICAL DATA ON REUSE 5
EDTA-ERA REGISTRY, Reuse Data 99, 101, 108
ENDOTOXINS 27, 29, 31, 66, 67, 71, 91
Cleaning Agent and 19
EOSINOPHILIA 158
ERYTHROCYTE, Survival of, Effect of Anti-N-Like Antibody 144
ESCHERICHIA COLI ENDOTOXIN 33
ESRD NETWORKS 184
ETHYLENE OXIDE 88, 145
Hypersensitivity Reactions 33
Toxicity 91
EUROPE see REUSE, by European Countries

FBV see FIBER BUNDLE VOLUME
FOOD AND DRUG ADMINISTRATION (FDA)
Guidelines for Reuse of Disposable Medical Devices—1977 93
Position on Reuse 184
FIBER BUNDLE VOLUME (FBV) 5, 19, 22, 77, 114, 167, 171, 194
Changes with Automated Reprocessing 173, 174
Comparison of Automated and Manual Determinations 173
Effect of Reuse on 40, 42
Initial Volume 82
Measurement of 28, 167
Relationship to Clearances 9
Relationship to Clearance of Small Molecules 118
Relationship to Membrane Area 5, 118
FIRST USE SYNDROME see NEW DIALYZER SYNDROME
FORMALDEHYDE ANALYSIS
Clinitest^R 4, 9, 22, 33, 140
Hantzsch Reaction 22,
Schiff's Reagent 120
Schiff's Reagent, Sensitivity 120
FORMALDEHYDE 4, 6, 21, 22, 29, 31, 51,

52, 65, 67, 111, 113, 114, 119, 140, 146, 187
Accidental I.V. Infusions 94
Analysis of, Spectrophotometric Determination 170
Asthma and 119
Binding to Dialyzer Membrane 142
Carcinogenesis and 57, 94, 119
Chemical Combination with Dialyzer Membrane 124
CDC Recommendations Regarding 6, 68, 70
Comparison with Other Disinfectants 70
Complement Activation in Treated Dialyzer 155
Contact Dermatitis and 119
Detection of 140, 141, 195
Patient Exposure to 146
Exposure to, Dialysis Personnel 86, 119
Hemolytic Anemia 94
Kinetics of Removal from Reused Dialyzers 52
Maximum Recommended Levels as Residual in Dialyzer 32
Methods for Detection 120
Nasal Squamous Cell Carcinomas in Animals 119
New Dialyzer Syndrome and 159
Preparation with Endotoxin Containing Water 71
Reaction with Dialyzer Membrane 124
Red Blood Cell Antibodies Induced by 135
Residual Concentration of, Effect on Anti-N-Like Antibody Formation 140, 147
Residual Dialyzer Levels, Effects of Different Flushing Methods 123, 142, 195
Residual Levels of 141
Spills 86
Toxicity 9, 91, 94
Use in Automated Reprocessing 164
Vapor Levels 86
FORMALERT^R 120
FORMOTEST^R 120

GLUTARALDEHYDE 29, 31, 111, 167, 170
Analysis of 34
Kinetics of Rinse Out 33

H_2O_2
Effectiveness as a Cleaning Agent 27
Use in Automated Reprocessing 166
HANTZSCH REACTION see FORMALDEHYDE ANALYSIS, HANTZSCH REACTION
HBsAG-POSITIVE PATIENTS 20
HCFA (HEALTH CARE FINANCING